Created by Xspurts.com

All rights reserved.

Copyright © 2005 onwards .

By reading this book, you agree to the below Terms and Conditions.

Xspurts.com retains all rights to these products.

No part of this book may be reproduced in any form, by photostat, microfilm, xerography, or any other means, or incorporated into any information retrieval system, electronic or mechanical, without the written permission of Xspurts.com; exceptions are made for brief excerpts used in published reviews.

This publication is designed to provide accurate and authoritative information with regard to the subject matter covered but is for entertainment purposes only. It is sold with the understanding that the publisher is not engaged in rendering legal, accounting, health, relationship or other professional / personal advice. If legal advice or other expert assistance is required, the services of a competent professional should be sought.

♥   A New Zealand Designed Product

Get A Free Book At: https://free.xspurts.com

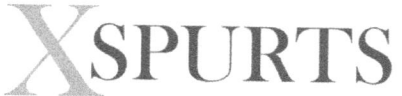

Table of Contents:

Table of Contents:
Understanding Ayurveda
Origin and Principles of Ayurveda
The Fundamental Concepts in Ayurveda
The Three Doshas
Ayurvedic Body Types
Vata, Pitta, Kapha Body Types
Determining Your Dosha
Balancing Your Doshas
Ayurveda and Nutrition
The Ayurvedic Diet
Ayurvedic Food Combinations and Recipes
Healing Herbs and Spices
Ayurveda and Detoxification
Purification Procedures in Ayurveda
Importance of Detoxification
Ayurvedic Home Remedies for Detox
Ayurveda and Yoga
Yoga Postures for Your Dosha
Ayurveda and Pranayama
Meditation Techniques in Ayurveda
Ayurvedic Daily Routine
Morning Rituals
Evening Practices
Seasonal Routines in Ayurveda
Ayurveda and Mental Health
Mind-Body Connection
Managing Stress with Ayurveda

- Ayurvedic Treatments for Mental Disorders
- Ayurveda and Sleep
- Ayurvedic Sleep Rituals
- Ayurvedic Remedies for Sleep Disorders
- Sleeping Positions in Ayurveda
- Ayurveda for Women
- Ayurveda and Female Health
- Ayurvedic Pregnancy Care
- Ayurveda and Menopause
- Ayurveda for Men
- Ayurveda for Male Vitality
- Ayurvedic Remedies for Common Men's Health Concerns
- Ayurveda and Beauty
- Ayurvedic Skin Care
- Natural Hair Care in Ayurveda
- Ayurvedic Oral Care
- Ayurveda and Aging
- Ayurvedic Approach to Aging
- Healthy Aging with Ayurveda
- Ayurvedic Herbs for Longevity
- Ayurvedic Treatments and Therapies
- Panchakarma - The Five Purification Procedures
- Ayurvedic Massages and Their Benefits
- Marma Therapy in Ayurveda
- Have Questions / Comments?
- Get Another Book Free

Understanding Ayurveda

Ayurveda is a holistic system of medicine that has been practiced for over 5,000 years in India. Its foundation rests on the belief that health and wellness are achieved through a balance between body, mind, and spirit, with an emphasis on the interconnectedness of all elements in the universe. The word "Ayurveda" comes from the Sanskrit terms "ayur," meaning life, and "veda," meaning knowledge or science. This ancient practice is based on the idea that everything in the universe, including the human body, is composed of five elements: earth, water, fire, air, and ether. These elements combine to form three primary energies or doshas: Vata, Pitta, and Kapha.

Each person has a unique constitution, or Prakriti, determined by the relative proportions of these doshas. When the doshas are balanced, the body and mind function optimally. However, imbalances—due to factors like diet, stress, environmental influences, or lifestyle choices—can lead to illness. Ayurveda aims to restore balance through personalized treatments that often include dietary changes, herbal remedies, meditation, yoga, and detoxification processes such as Panchakarma.

The doshas play a central role in diagnosing and treating conditions in Ayurveda. Vata is linked to movement and is responsible for functions like circulation, respiration, and communication within the body. Pitta governs metabolism, digestion, and transformation. Kapha is associated with structure, immunity, and fluid balance. Each individual's dosha composition is assessed to create a treatment plan that aligns with their unique needs and lifestyle.

One of the cornerstones of Ayurvedic practice is the idea of food as medicine. A diet tailored to an individual's dosha type can help maintain harmony within the body. For example, a person with a dominant Pitta dosha might be advised to consume cooling foods to counteract the heating nature of Pitta, while someone with a Kapha imbalance might benefit from light, dry foods to stimulate digestion and metabolism.

Ayurveda also emphasizes the importance of mental and emotional well-being in overall health. Meditation, breathing exercises (pranayama), and yoga are integral components of the practice, aimed at calming the mind, reducing stress, and promoting clarity. These practices not only complement the physical treatments but also enhance the body's ability to heal.

Herbal remedies are a key aspect of Ayurvedic medicine. Plants, herbs, and minerals are used in precise formulations to treat a wide range of ailments. Some herbs, like Ashwagandha, Turmeric, and Triphala, are widely known for their adaptogenic, anti-inflammatory, and detoxifying properties, respectively. Ayurvedic practitioners believe that these natural substances work in harmony with the body's energies to restore balance and health.

The practice of Ayurveda is personalized and holistic, considering the body's physical, emotional, and spiritual needs. Its comprehensive approach has attracted growing attention worldwide as people seek alternative and complementary healing methods that promote long-term wellness rather than just symptom management. By embracing the principles of balance and prevention, Ayurveda offers a unique perspective on maintaining health that aligns with nature's rhythms and the individual's inherent constitution.

Origin and Principles of Ayurveda

The origins of Ayurveda can be traced back to ancient India, where it is considered one of the oldest systems of medicine in the world. Its roots are deeply embedded in Vedic traditions, with the earliest texts dating back to around 1500 BCE. The knowledge of Ayurveda was passed down orally through generations and was eventually written down in sacred texts known as the "Vedas," particularly the Atharvaveda. Over time, these teachings evolved into a comprehensive system of health and healing, focusing on the prevention and treatment of disease through natural means.

The core principles of Ayurveda revolve around the concept of balance, both within the body and in relation to the environment. At its heart, Ayurveda believes that the universe is made up of five basic elements—earth, water, fire, air, and ether—which combine in various ways to form three primary energies or doshas: Vata, Pitta, and Kapha. Each dosha governs specific functions and processes in the body and mind.

Vata is associated with movement and is responsible for bodily functions such as breathing, circulation, and communication between cells. Pitta, linked to the fire element, controls digestion, metabolism, and transformation. Kapha, connected to the earth and water elements, governs structure, stability, and immunity. Each individual is believed to have a unique constitution, or Prakriti, which is a specific combination of these doshas, and the balance of these energies is key to maintaining health.

When the doshas are in harmony, the body operates optimally, but an imbalance—caused by factors like poor diet, stress, environmental influences, or lifestyle choices—can lead to illness or disease. Ayurveda emphasizes that health is not simply the absence of disease but a state of complete physical, mental, and spiritual well-being. As such, it focuses not just on treating symptoms but on addressing the root cause of health problems by restoring balance to the body's energies.

The guiding philosophy of Ayurveda encourages prevention over treatment. This means adopting daily habits (Dinacharya) and seasonal routines (Ritucharya) that align with the body's natural rhythms and the cycles of nature. These practices include mindful eating, exercise, rest, and self-care, all of which contribute to long-term well-being. Ayurveda also emphasizes the importance of digestion, or Agni, which is considered the cornerstone of good health. A strong digestive fire leads to proper absorption of nutrients, while weak digestion is thought to result in toxins (Ama) accumulating in the body, potentially leading to disease.

In treatment, Ayurveda takes a holistic approach that considers not only the physical body but also the emotional and spiritual aspects of a person. Herbal remedies, detoxification (Panchakarma), yoga, and meditation are commonly used to restore balance and promote healing. Unlike conventional medicine, which often targets specific symptoms, Ayurveda seeks to harmonize the body, mind, and spirit, ensuring a person's overall vitality and longevity.

By viewing health as a dynamic interplay between the individual and their environment, Ayurveda offers a timeless approach to wellness that remains relevant today, offering a path to living in harmony with nature and the self.

The Fundamental Concepts in Ayurveda

At the heart of Ayurveda are several fundamental concepts that form the framework of its practice and philosophy. These concepts reflect the holistic nature of the system, emphasizing balance, interconnectedness, and the body's ability to heal itself. Understanding these principles helps clarify how Ayurveda addresses health and well-being on a deep, individualized level.

One of the key concepts is **the five elements**—earth, water, fire, air, and ether—often referred to as *Pancha Mahabhutas*. These elements are believed to make up all matter in the universe, including the human body. Each element corresponds to particular physical and mental functions. Earth provides structure and stability, water governs fluids and lubrication, fire relates to transformation and digestion, air is responsible for movement and circulation, and ether represents space and consciousness. The balance of these elements within the body determines overall health.

These five elements combine to form the **three doshas**, which are the biological energies that govern bodily functions. **Vata**, composed of air and ether, is responsible for movement, including breathing, circulation, and nerve impulses. **Pitta**, made up of fire and water, governs metabolism, digestion, and transformation processes. **Kapha**, a combination of earth and water, oversees structure, growth, and immunity. Each person has a unique combination of these doshas, known as their **Prakriti**, which influences their physical characteristics, mental state, and susceptibility to illness.

When the doshas are in harmony, the body and mind are healthy. However, if these energies become imbalanced due to external factors such as poor diet, stress, or environmental changes, it can lead to disease. Ayurveda views illness as the result of an imbalance in the doshas and seeks to restore equilibrium through personalized treatments.

Another central concept in Ayurveda is **Agni**, or the digestive fire. According to Ayurvedic belief, digestion is the foundation of health, and a strong Agni is essential for the proper absorption of nutrients and elimination of waste. When Agni is weak, food is not properly digested, leading to the accumulation of undigested material or **Ama**. Ama is considered the root cause of disease in Ayurveda, as it can accumulate in the tissues and block the flow of vital energy (Prana), leading to toxicity and illness.

The concept of **Ojas** is closely linked to the idea of vitality and immunity. Ojas represents the essence of physical strength, mental clarity, and emotional stability. It is the byproduct of proper digestion and balanced doshas and is thought to govern immunity and the body's ability to resist disease. When Ojas is abundant, a person feels energetic, mentally sharp, and emotionally balanced.

Dhatus are the seven tissues of the body, and they include plasma, blood, muscles, fat, bone, marrow, and reproductive tissue. The health of these tissues is directly influenced by the strength of Agni and the balance of the doshas. Ayurveda emphasizes nourishing and cleansing these tissues to maintain vitality and prevent disease.

In addition to these physical principles, Ayurveda also underscores the importance of **mind-body connection**. The emotional and mental state of an individual plays a crucial role in overall health. Practices like meditation, pranayama (breathing exercises), and yoga are used to cultivate mental clarity, reduce stress, and enhance emotional well-being. Ayurveda sees the mind as a powerful influence on the body and promotes techniques to calm the mind and nurture emotional health.

Ultimately, the goal of Ayurveda is not just to treat disease but to promote a state of balance and harmony within the individual, ensuring a life of vitality and well-being. Its principles offer a comprehensive approach to health that considers the unique nature of each person and the intricate relationship between body, mind, and spirit. Through the application of Ayurvedic concepts, individuals can achieve a state of lasting wellness that aligns with the rhythms of nature.

The Three Doshas

In Ayurveda, the three doshas—Vata, Pitta, and Kapha—are fundamental energies believed to govern the physical and mental processes of the body. These doshas are derived from the five elements—earth, water, fire, air, and ether—and each dosha is a unique combination of these elements, influencing everything from bodily functions to emotional states. Each person is thought to have a specific balance of these doshas that defines their unique constitution, known as **Prakriti**.

Vata is the dosha primarily associated with movement and change. It is a combination of air and ether, and it governs functions such as breathing, circulation, nerve impulses, and elimination. Vata controls the nervous system, the body's ability to move and adapt, and the processes of creativity and communication. People with a dominant Vata dosha tend to be energetic, quick-thinking, and adaptable. However, when out of balance, Vata can cause restlessness, anxiety, digestive irregularities, and dry skin. Physically, those with a Vata constitution may have a slender frame, dry skin, and colder body temperature.

Pitta is associated with transformation, heat, and metabolism. It is composed of fire and water and governs digestion, absorption, metabolism, and body temperature. Pitta is responsible for converting food into energy, managing the body's internal heat, and regulating the hormonal and enzymatic functions. Those with a strong Pitta influence tend to be determined, focused, and competitive. They may be prone to becoming overheated, both physically and emotionally, and are more susceptible to conditions like inflammation, acidity, and stress-related disorders when Pitta is out of balance. Individuals with a Pitta constitution generally have a medium build, warm body temperature, and may be prone to sensitive skin or rashes.

Kapha, composed of earth and water, governs structure, stability, and lubrication. It is responsible for maintaining the body's strength, immunity, and fluid balance. Kapha provides the body with physical structure and support, including the health of the bones, tissues, and joints. It also helps in the formation of bodily fluids such as mucus and saliva. People with a dominant Kapha dosha are often calm, patient, and nurturing, with strong endurance and a tendency to be more grounded. When Kapha becomes imbalanced, however, it can lead to weight gain, sluggish digestion, congestion, and excessive mucus production. Those with a Kapha constitution often have a sturdy, well-built frame, smooth skin, and a tendency to retain water.

In Ayurveda, the health of an individual is determined by the balance of these doshas. When they are in harmony, the body and mind function optimally, but when one or more doshas become imbalanced, it can lead to physical and mental ailments. Treatment in Ayurveda is personalized based on a person's unique doshic constitution and the specific imbalance they may be experiencing. By understanding the doshas and their effects on the body and mind, Ayurveda provides a pathway to health that promotes equilibrium and well-being.

Ayurvedic Body Types

In Ayurveda, each individual has a unique constitution, or **Prakriti**, that is determined by the balance of the three doshas—Vata, Pitta, and Kapha. This constitution dictates not only physical traits but also mental and emotional characteristics. Understanding one's Ayurvedic body type can offer valuable insights into health, diet, and lifestyle choices, as it helps tailor practices and habits that align with the natural rhythms of the body. These body types are categorized based on the predominant dosha, and each comes with distinct qualities.

Vata Body Type
A person with a dominant Vata dosha tends to have a lighter frame with angular features. Their body is typically slim, with dry skin, and they often have a lower body temperature. Vata types are usually active, energetic, and creative, but they can also be prone to instability, restlessness, and dryness in both the body and mind. Their digestion may be irregular, and they often experience a quick metabolism. Mentally, they are quick thinkers, imaginative, and adaptable, but may struggle with anxiety or a tendency to overthink. A balanced Vata body type will have good circulation and flexibility, but when imbalanced, they may experience conditions like insomnia, digestive issues, or mood swings. Vata individuals benefit from regular routines, warm foods, and practices that ground and calm the mind, such as yoga and meditation.

Pitta Body Type
Pitta-dominant individuals are typically medium-built with a well-defined physique. They have warm, oily skin and a strong appetite. Pitta types tend to be ambitious, focused, and intelligent, with a natural ability to lead. They excel in high-pressure situations and are often goal-driven. Physically, they have good muscle tone and a strong digestion, but can be prone to conditions related to excess heat, such as inflammation, acidity, and rashes. Mentally, Pitta types are sharp and can be intense or even prone to irritability when imbalanced. They may suffer from stress and frustration if their needs for achievement and control are not met. To maintain balance, Pitta types should adopt cooling practices, such as spending time in nature, eating cooling foods like fruits and leafy greens, and avoiding excessive heat or anger-triggering situations.

Kapha Body Type
Kapha individuals generally have a larger, well-built body with rounded features. They are typically strong, sturdy, and have a slower metabolism. Kapha types have thick, smooth skin and tend to retain moisture and body weight more easily. Emotionally, they

are calm, stable, and compassionate, with an ability to nurture and care for others. However, when imbalanced, Kapha types can become lethargic, overattached, or overly possessive. They may experience weight gain, congestion, and digestive sluggishness. Mentally, Kapha types are patient and grounded but may struggle with mental heaviness or depression when out of balance. For Kapha individuals, maintaining an active lifestyle, eating lighter foods, and incorporating invigorating activities like walking or vigorous yoga can help balance excess Kapha energy.

Each person's constitution is a blend of these doshas, with one or two doshas typically being more dominant. For example, a person might be predominantly Vata with some Pitta traits, or a balanced mix of all three doshas. Ayurveda holds that understanding your body type is key to finding the right diet, exercise, and lifestyle to maintain health. By recognizing the characteristics of your Ayurvedic body type, you can cultivate better habits and achieve greater harmony in both body and mind.

Vata, Pitta, Kapha Body Types

In Ayurveda, each individual is believed to have a unique combination of the three doshas—Vata, Pitta, and Kapha—forming a distinctive body type. These doshas govern various physical, mental, and emotional characteristics, and understanding one's doshic makeup can provide valuable insights into maintaining health and well-being. Each dosha represents a specific set of qualities, and the body type associated with each dosha exhibits distinct traits that influence a person's overall constitution.

Vata Body Type
Vata types are characterized by their light, thin, and often delicate build. Their body tends to have angular features, and they may have dry skin and a cooler body temperature. People with a dominant Vata dosha are typically quick-moving, energetic, and creative, often with a restless or spontaneous nature. Vata types may experience irregular digestion, with fluctuating appetite and tendency toward bloating or gas. Mentally, they are imaginative, flexible, and have a rapid thought process, though they can also be prone to anxiety, overthinking, and instability when Vata is out of balance. Those with a Vata constitution benefit from warmth and routine—warm foods, regular sleep, and calming practices like yoga and meditation help to maintain balance. When imbalanced, they may suffer from conditions like insomnia, dry skin, or digestive disorders.

Pitta Body Type
Individuals with a dominant Pitta dosha typically have a medium or muscular build with a strong, well-defined body. They have oily skin, a warm body temperature, and often have a robust appetite. Pitta types are known for their sharp intellect, determination, and strong will. They excel in leadership roles, thriving in competitive environments, but they can also become irritable or impatient if their needs are not met. Pitta types tend to have a strong digestion, but if imbalanced, they may experience conditions related to heat, such as acidity, inflammation, or skin rashes. Mentally, they are focused and goal-oriented but can become overly intense or prone to anger when Pitta becomes excessive. To maintain balance, Pitta types should incorporate cooling, calming practices like spending time in nature, eating cooling foods (such as fruits and leafy vegetables), and avoiding extreme heat or stress.

Kapha Body Type
Kapha types generally have a larger, sturdier build with rounded features. They often have smooth, oily skin and a slower metabolism. People with a dominant Kapha dosha tend to be calm, patient, and nurturing, with a strong sense of stability and endurance.

Kapha individuals are known for their ability to retain water and build muscle mass, but they may also be prone to weight gain, sluggish digestion, and excess mucus production when imbalanced. Mentally, Kapha types are grounded and steady, but they can become overly attached, resistant to change, or prone to feelings of lethargy and heaviness when out of balance. To maintain equilibrium, Kapha types benefit from regular physical activity, lighter foods, and practices that invigorate the body and mind, such as stimulating yoga or engaging in social activities.

Understanding these body types allows for a more personalized approach to health and wellness. Each person's constitution, or **Prakriti**, is a unique blend of the doshas, with one or two doshas often being more dominant. By recognizing and respecting these inherent qualities, Ayurveda encourages individuals to make lifestyle choices that align with their dosha, fostering harmony and vitality. Whether it's adjusting diet, exercise routines, or mindfulness practices, Ayurveda provides a guide to living in tune with one's natural body type.

Determining Your Dosha

In Ayurveda, determining your dosha is an essential step toward understanding your body's unique constitution and achieving optimal health. The three doshas—Vata, Pitta, and Kapha—represent different energies in the body, each with its own characteristics that influence physical, mental, and emotional well-being. Everyone has a primary dosha, but most people also have a secondary dosha or a combination of doshas that help define their overall constitution. By assessing various factors, such as your physical traits, temperament, and health patterns, you can identify your dominant dosha and gain insights into how to balance your body and mind.

Physical Characteristics
Your body's build and appearance can offer important clues about your dosha. **Vata** types typically have a slender, lean frame with dry skin and cold hands and feet. They may have prominent bones and a light, agile physique. **Pitta** types tend to have a medium, muscular build with warm, oily skin. Their features are often sharp, and they may have a strong appetite and quick metabolism. **Kapha** types are generally sturdy with a round or stocky build. They have smooth, soft skin and may be prone to weight gain and fluid retention.

Mental and Emotional Traits
Each dosha influences your mental and emotional tendencies as well. **Vata** individuals are often energetic, creative, and quick-thinking but can also be prone to anxiety, restlessness, and nervousness. **Pitta** types are driven, focused, and sharp-minded, with a natural ability to lead. However, they can become irritable, competitive, or prone to anger when out of balance. **Kapha** types are calm, compassionate, and patient, often enjoying stability and routine. When out of balance, they may become overly attached, sluggish, or prone to depression.

Health Patterns
Your health and susceptibility to certain conditions also point to your dosha. **Vata** types may experience irregular digestion, bloating, and dry skin. They tend to feel cold easily and may suffer from anxiety or insomnia. **Pitta** individuals typically have strong digestion and a robust appetite but may be prone to digestive issues like acid reflux or heartburn, as well as inflammation or skin rashes. **Kapha** types often experience slower digestion and may be prone to excess mucus, weight gain, or conditions like allergies or congestion.

Lifestyle Preferences

Your lifestyle habits and preferences can also indicate your dosha. **Vata** types enjoy variety, spontaneity, and creative expression. They may struggle with maintaining routine and can feel overwhelmed by excessive activity. **Pitta** individuals thrive on structure and productivity, often pursuing high-achieving goals. They enjoy challenge but need to avoid excessive stress or overwork. **Kapha** types prefer calm environments and often enjoy stability and consistency. They may find it difficult to adapt to change but excel in nurturing and caring roles.

How to Determine Your Dosha

To determine your dosha, Ayurvedic practitioners often assess your physical features, personality traits, emotional tendencies, and health history. While this can be done through questionnaires or consultations with an Ayurvedic expert, you can also do it by carefully observing yourself over time. Pay attention to your body's tendencies, your moods, and your reactions to various environments, foods, and routines.

In addition to these personal observations, Ayurveda also considers the current state of your doshas. You might have a dominant dosha, but an imbalance in one of the other doshas can influence your current health state. For example, a Vata imbalance might result in dry skin and anxiety, while a Pitta imbalance could lead to inflammation and irritability.

Balancing Your Dosha

Once you have an understanding of your dosha, Ayurveda offers guidance on how to keep it balanced. This may involve dietary recommendations, lifestyle adjustments, and specific practices that harmonize your doshic energies. For example, **Vata types** benefit from grounding, warm foods and calming routines. **Pitta types** should focus on cooling foods, stress-reduction techniques, and maintaining a balance between work and rest. **Kapha types** thrive with stimulating activities, light foods, and a dynamic lifestyle to prevent stagnation.

By identifying your dosha and understanding its characteristics, you can create a personalized approach to health that aligns with your unique constitution. This knowledge not only helps prevent disease but also fosters a sense of balance and vitality in your daily life.

Balancing Your Doshas

In Ayurveda, balancing the doshas is essential for maintaining overall health and well-being. Each of the three doshas—Vata, Pitta, and Kapha—has distinct characteristics, and when one or more of them become imbalanced, it can lead to physical, mental, and emotional disturbances. Achieving balance involves aligning your diet, lifestyle, and habits with your dominant dosha or the current state of imbalance. The goal is to bring harmony to the body's energies, preventing illness and fostering vitality.

Balancing Vata
Vata, the dosha associated with air and ether, is responsible for movement and communication within the body. When Vata becomes imbalanced, it can lead to dryness, anxiety, and irregular digestion. To balance Vata, focus on grounding, stabilizing practices that soothe its light and erratic nature.

Diet plays a key role in calming Vata. Warm, nourishing foods like soups, stews, and cooked grains help counteract Vata's dry, cold qualities. Choose foods that are sweet, sour, or salty to balance the lightness of Vata—avoid raw or cold foods, as they can aggravate the dosha. **Vata types** should also prioritize routine, ensuring regular sleep patterns and eating habits, as unpredictability can worsen imbalances.

Lifestyle practices for balancing Vata include stress reduction and grounding activities. Regular yoga, particularly slow, gentle poses, and meditation can calm the nervous system and promote relaxation. Staying warm in both body and environment also helps balance Vata's cool tendencies. Additionally, limiting exposure to excessive stimulation or busy environments is key to maintaining calm and focus.

Balancing Pitta
Pitta, made up of fire and water, governs metabolism, digestion, and transformation. When Pitta is out of balance, it can lead to irritability, inflammation, acidity, and skin rashes. To restore balance, focus on cooling, soothing practices that counteract Pitta's hot, intense nature.

Pitta types should emphasize cooling foods, such as cucumbers, leafy greens, dairy, and sweet fruits. Foods that are bitter, astringent, and sweet are ideal for calming Pitta, while hot, spicy, and sour foods should be minimized. Eating smaller, more frequent meals can help maintain digestive health and prevent overheating.

Stress reduction is crucial for balancing Pitta. Practices like mindfulness, deep breathing, and spending time in nature help calm the fire element. It's important for **Pitta types** to avoid overexertion, particularly in hot environments, and to allow for plenty of rest and relaxation to prevent burnout. Gentle exercise like swimming, walking, or light yoga is beneficial, but high-intensity workouts should be avoided to prevent excessive heat from building up in the body.

Balancing Kapha
Kapha, the dosha of earth and water, is responsible for structure, stability, and immunity. When Kapha is imbalanced, it can lead to sluggish digestion, weight gain, and feelings of heaviness or lethargy. To bring Kapha into balance, it's important to stimulate and invigorate the body and mind.

For Kapha, a light, dry, and warm diet is ideal. Avoid heavy, oily foods like fried or processed items, and focus on foods that are spicy, bitter, and astringent to help stimulate digestion. Foods like beans, vegetables, and whole grains are perfect for balancing Kapha. Regular fasting or lighter meals can help prevent sluggishness.

Exercise is essential for balancing Kapha, and more vigorous physical activity is beneficial. Aerobic exercises, such as running, cycling, or vigorous yoga, are excellent for promoting circulation and energy. Kapha types should also engage in activities that break their routine and challenge them mentally, avoiding the tendency to become too comfortable or stuck in a rut.

Mental stimulation and social engagement are also helpful for balancing Kapha, as it prevents the tendency toward attachment or depression. Practices that encourage movement and flexibility in both body and mind, such as dance or creative expression, can lift the heavy energy that Kapha can bring.

General Tips for Balancing the Doshas
In addition to dosha-specific recommendations, Ayurveda emphasizes the importance of aligning with nature's rhythms. This includes following a daily routine (*Dinacharya*) that supports health—waking up early, eating meals at consistent times, and getting adequate rest. Seasonal routines (*Ritucharya*) also play a role, as each season influences the doshas. For example, during the cold and dry winter months, Vata may become aggravated, requiring extra care in keeping warm and nourished.

Self-care rituals, such as oil massages (*Abhyanga*), herbal teas, and detoxifying treatments, also support the balancing of doshas. Ayurveda encourages a lifestyle that fosters a connection between the mind, body, and spirit, focusing on preventive care and long-term wellness rather than merely treating symptoms.

By understanding your dosha and implementing these practices, you can achieve greater harmony and prevent the onset of disease. Ayurveda's holistic approach encourages you to listen to your body and make conscious choices to nurture your health and balance throughout life.

Ayurveda and Nutrition

In Ayurveda, nutrition is not just about what you eat, but also how, when, and why you eat. Ayurveda views food as medicine, and emphasizes the importance of a balanced, personalized diet that aligns with an individual's unique constitution, or dosha. The goal is to nourish the body, mind, and spirit while promoting overall health, vitality, and longevity. Food is considered a key element in balancing the doshas, and Ayurveda suggests that the right foods can prevent illness and promote wellness when consumed in harmony with the body's needs.

The principles of Ayurvedic nutrition are deeply rooted in the concept of digestion, or **Agni**. Agni, often referred to as the "digestive fire," is central to the Ayurvedic approach to food and health. When Agni is strong, the body is able to properly digest food, absorb nutrients, and eliminate waste. However, when Agni is weak or imbalanced, the body may struggle to digest food effectively, leading to the buildup of toxins (*Ama*) that can cause disease. Thus, the focus in Ayurveda is on optimizing digestion and ensuring that the food you eat supports your body's natural processes.

Food Choices Based on Dosha
Each of the three doshas—Vata, Pitta, and Kapha—has specific dietary needs. The foods that balance one dosha might aggravate another, so understanding your constitution helps guide dietary choices.

- **Vata:** Since Vata is characterized by dryness, coldness, and lightness, those with a predominant Vata dosha benefit from warm, moist, and grounding foods. Sweet, sour, and salty flavors help to calm the erratic nature of Vata. Foods like cooked grains, root vegetables, soups, and stews are ideal. Vata types should avoid raw foods, cold drinks, and overly bitter or astringent flavors, as these can aggravate the dosha and disturb digestion.
- **Pitta:** Pitta types, associated with heat and intensity, thrive on cooling and soothing foods. Pitta is balanced by sweet, bitter, and astringent flavors, while spicy, sour, and salty foods should be minimized. Fresh fruits, leafy greens, and dairy products like milk and yogurt are beneficial for calming Pitta. Pitta individuals should avoid foods that are too hot, spicy, or fried, as these can increase their internal heat and cause issues like acidity or inflammation.
- **Kapha:** Kapha types, known for their stability and heaviness, benefit from light, dry, and stimulating foods. Spicy, bitter, and astringent flavors help to balance Kapha, while heavy, oily, and sweet foods should be reduced. Foods such as

legumes, vegetables, and whole grains are ideal for Kapha types. Kapha types are also advised to limit dairy and cold foods, as these can increase mucus production and lead to sluggish digestion.

The Importance of Food Timing

In Ayurveda, when you eat is just as important as what you eat. It is believed that eating at the right time enhances the body's ability to digest and absorb nutrients. For optimal digestion, it's recommended to eat the largest meal of the day at lunch, when digestive fire is strongest. Light meals should be consumed in the evening, and dinner should ideally be eaten at least two to three hours before bedtime.

Ayurveda also advises eating in a calm, mindful state to support digestion. Eating in a relaxed environment without distractions such as television or stress helps activate the body's parasympathetic nervous system, which promotes digestion. Additionally, it is recommended to avoid drinking large amounts of water during meals, as this can dilute digestive juices and hinder proper digestion.

The Role of Spices and Herbs

Spices and herbs play a central role in Ayurvedic nutrition, not only enhancing flavor but also supporting digestion and health. Many common kitchen spices have medicinal properties that aid in the digestion of food, balance the doshas, and detoxify the body. For example, **turmeric** is known for its anti-inflammatory properties, **ginger** stimulates digestion, and **cumin** and **fennel** support healthy digestion and metabolism.

Herbs such as **Triphala**, **Ashwagandha**, and **Tulsi** (holy basil) are frequently used in Ayurvedic medicine to promote overall health, improve digestion, and balance the doshas. Ayurvedic practitioners often recommend herbal teas made with ingredients like ginger, peppermint, or cardamom to soothe the digestive system and enhance digestion.

Food and Lifestyle Integration

In addition to focusing on food itself, Ayurveda encourages integrating lifestyle habits that support overall health. A balanced routine that includes regular exercise, adequate rest, and stress management is just as important as the food you eat. Ayurveda also emphasizes the importance of mindful eating—taking the time to chew food thoroughly and savor each bite to improve digestion and absorption.

The Ayurvedic approach to nutrition is highly personalized, taking into account not only your dosha but also seasonal changes, age, and lifestyle factors. For example, during the colder months, heavier and warmer foods are recommended to balance the cold and dry qualities of the season, while in warmer months, lighter and cooling foods are advised to counteract the heat.

Ultimately, Ayurveda teaches that nutrition is a dynamic and integral part of overall health, with food serving as a bridge between the body and mind. By making mindful choices that are in harmony with your body's unique needs, you can nourish yourself on all levels—physically, mentally, and spiritually—leading to a balanced and vibrant life.

The Ayurvedic Diet

In Ayurveda, diet is considered a fundamental pillar of health and well-being. The Ayurvedic diet emphasizes balance, digestion, and nourishment, recognizing that food is not just fuel, but medicine for the body, mind, and spirit. Unlike conventional approaches to nutrition that often focus on calorie counts or specific nutrients, Ayurveda seeks to align your diet with your unique constitution (Prakriti), the changing seasons, and the current state of balance or imbalance in your body (Vikriti). The focus is on creating harmony between the body's internal environment and the external world to maintain optimal health.

The Importance of Agni (Digestive Fire)
In Ayurveda, digestion is paramount. The concept of **Agni**, or digestive fire, is central to understanding the Ayurvedic approach to food. Strong Agni is necessary for proper digestion, absorption of nutrients, and elimination of waste. When Agni is weak, food is poorly digested, leading to the formation of **Ama**, a toxic substance that can cause disease. A healthy diet in Ayurveda is designed to nourish and strengthen Agni, ensuring that food is properly digested and utilized by the body.

Diet According to Dosha
Each individual has a dominant dosha—Vata, Pitta, or Kapha—that influences both physical and mental characteristics. Ayurveda believes that dietary recommendations should be tailored to your dosha to maintain balance. For example:

- **Vata** types, who tend to be light, dry, and cold, benefit from warm, moist, and grounding foods. Sweet, salty, and sour tastes help balance Vata. Foods like soups, stews, cooked grains, and root vegetables are ideal. Vata individuals should avoid raw, dry, or cold foods, as these can aggravate their constitution.
- **Pitta** types, characterized by heat, sharpness, and intensity, are cooled by sweet, bitter, and astringent tastes. Foods such as leafy greens, cucumbers, dairy products, and cooling fruits like melons help to soothe Pitta. Spicy, sour, and oily foods should be minimized to prevent excess heat from building up.
- **Kapha** types, with their heavy, stable, and moist qualities, benefit from light, dry, and stimulating foods. Spicy, bitter, and astringent flavors help balance Kapha, while sweet, salty, and oily foods should be avoided. Kapha types thrive on vegetables, legumes, and grains that are light and easy to digest.

The Six Tastes (Shad Rasa)

In Ayurveda, the **six tastes**—sweet, sour, salty, bitter, pungent, and astringent—are thought to have specific effects on the doshas. These tastes are not only enjoyed for flavor but also for their therapeutic properties. A balanced Ayurvedic meal includes all six tastes to ensure that the body receives a range of nutrients and to create harmony between the doshas.

- **Sweet** foods, such as grains, fruits, and dairy, nourish the body and calm Vata.
- **Sour** foods, like citrus and fermented items, stimulate digestion and balance Kapha.
- **Salty** foods, found in salt and sea vegetables, support digestion and help reduce dehydration.
- **Bitter** tastes, present in leafy greens and herbs like turmeric, help detoxify and balance Pitta.
- **Pungent** foods, such as spicy peppers and garlic, increase circulation and stimulate digestion.
- **Astringent** foods, like legumes and pomegranate, help absorb excess moisture and are useful for Kapha types.

Seasonal and Circadian Rhythms

Ayurveda stresses the importance of eating in harmony with the seasons and the body's internal rhythms. **Seasonal eating** encourages consuming foods that align with the environment. For example, during the cold winter months, warming, grounding foods are recommended, such as soups, root vegetables, and stews. In the heat of summer, lighter, cooling foods like salads, fruits, and dairy are favored.

Similarly, Ayurvedic principles recommend eating according to the time of day to match the body's natural cycles. The largest meal should be consumed at lunch, when digestion is strongest (between 12 PM and 2 PM), while a lighter dinner should be eaten early in the evening to allow proper digestion before bedtime. Ayurveda also recommends eating mindfully and chewing food thoroughly to aid digestion.

The Role of Spices and Herbs

Spices and herbs play an integral role in the Ayurvedic diet, not just for flavor but also for their medicinal properties. Spices like **turmeric, ginger, cumin,** and **fennel** are used to stimulate digestion, reduce inflammation, and balance the doshas. Herbal teas made from ingredients such as **mint, chamomile,** and **coriander** are commonly used to soothe the digestive system, promote detoxification, and calm the mind.

Eating Mindfully

Mindful eating is an essential practice in Ayurveda. It's believed that the mind should be calm and focused while eating to support proper digestion. Ayurveda recommends eating in a relaxed environment, free from distractions like television or stressful situations, to help activate the body's parasympathetic nervous system. This promotes the production of digestive enzymes, improving the body's ability to absorb nutrients and eliminate waste.

The Ayurvedic diet emphasizes food that is nourishing, balanced, and in alignment with your body's unique needs. By considering your dosha, eating with the seasons, and focusing on digestive health, Ayurveda encourages a holistic approach to nutrition that fosters overall well-being. Whether it's through the therapeutic use of spices, mindful eating practices, or personalized dietary recommendations, Ayurveda teaches that food is not just fuel but an essential part of the body's healing and balance.

Ayurvedic Food Combinations and Recipes

In Ayurveda, food combinations play a critical role in promoting optimal digestion and health. Ayurvedic principles suggest that certain foods, when combined, can enhance the body's ability to absorb nutrients and maintain balance, while others, when paired incorrectly, can disrupt digestion and cause imbalances. The key to Ayurvedic food combinations is harmonizing tastes, qualities, and energies of different foods, ensuring they complement each other and support the body's digestive fire, or **Agni**.

Principles of Ayurvedic Food Combinations
In Ayurveda, it's essential to combine foods based on their properties, which include taste, temperature, and effect on the doshas. There are a few general guidelines for healthy food combinations:

- **Avoid combining dairy with meat**: This combination can be difficult for the body to digest and can lead to the production of toxins (Ama).
- **Do not mix fruits with other foods**: Fruits are best eaten on their own, as they digest quickly and can interfere with the digestion of heavier foods.
- **Limit combining proteins and starches**: Ayurvedic tradition suggests that proteins (like meat, beans, and lentils) should not be eaten with heavy starches (like potatoes, rice, or bread), as they require different digestive enzymes and can create sluggish digestion.
- **Pair warm foods with cooling foods**: Combining warming spices (like ginger or garlic) with cooling foods (like cucumber or dairy) can balance heat and help digestion.
- **Use spices to aid digestion**: Spices are considered essential for boosting Agni and aiding digestion. Incorporating ingredients like cumin, coriander, turmeric, and ginger helps stimulate digestive fire and improve nutrient absorption.

Ayurvedic Food Combinations for Different Doshas
Each dosha requires specific food combinations that support its inherent qualities. Balancing the doshas through diet can help promote health and prevent imbalances.

- **Vata**: For the airy and dry qualities of Vata, grounding and moisturizing foods are needed. **Warm stews**, **soups**, and **root vegetables** are ideal for Vata. Combining **sweet** and **salty** tastes with **healthy fats** such as ghee or olive oil works well. For example, a **sweet potato stew with ghee, cumin, and coriander** can be both soothing and satisfying. Vata types also benefit from **spicy soups** like **ginger and turmeric soup**, which help stimulate digestion and keep Vata's erratic energy grounded.

- **Pitta**: Since Pitta is fiery and intense, Pitta types require cooling foods to keep the internal heat balanced. **Cool salads**, **leafy greens**, and **cucumber** pair well with **sweet** and **bitter** flavors. A **cucumber mint raita** made with yogurt, cucumber, mint, and cumin is a refreshing combination that cools Pitta while aiding digestion. A **Pitta-balancing salad** made with mixed greens, avocado, and a light lemon dressing offers cooling and soothing qualities to counterbalance Pitta's heat.
- **Kapha**: Kapha types, known for their slow metabolism and tendency to retain weight, benefit from stimulating, light, and spicy foods. Spices like **black pepper**, **mustard**, and **ginger** help enhance digestion. **Spicy lentil soup** made with turmeric, garlic, and ginger can boost metabolism and stimulate digestion. Combining **bitter greens** like **kale** or **spinach** with **spicy chutneys** or a tangy **tomato and mustard sauce** can energize Kapha and prevent sluggishness.

Ayurvedic Recipes

1. **Kitchari** – A traditional Ayurvedic dish that combines rice and lentils, providing a gentle cleanse for the body. It's a balanced meal that can be tailored to each dosha with specific spices.

   Ingredients:
   - 1/2 cup basmati rice
   - 1/4 cup mung dal (yellow split lentils)
   - 1 tablespoon ghee
   - 1 teaspoon cumin seeds
   - 1/2 teaspoon turmeric powder
   - 1/4 teaspoon coriander powder
   - Salt to taste
   - 4 cups water
   - Fresh cilantro for garnish

   Method:
   10. Wash the rice and mung dal thoroughly and set aside.
   11. Heat the ghee in a pot and add cumin seeds. Let them sizzle for a few seconds, then add the turmeric and coriander powders.
   12. Add the rice and dal mixture to the pot, stir for a few minutes, and then add water.

13. Bring the mixture to a boil, then reduce heat and simmer for 20–30 minutes until the rice and lentils are soft.
14. Season with salt and garnish with fresh cilantro. Serve warm.

This dish is soothing and nourishing, especially good for balancing Vata and Kapha doshas. Pitta types can adjust by omitting the chili peppers and adding cooling ingredients like coconut.

2. **Cooling Pitta Salad with Avocado and Cucumber** – A light, refreshing salad that cools internal heat and provides hydration.

Ingredients:

- 1 cucumber, sliced
- 1 ripe avocado, diced
- 1 tablespoon fresh lemon juice
- 1 teaspoon olive oil
- Fresh cilantro, chopped
- Salt and black pepper to taste
- A pinch of ground cumin

Method:

8. In a large bowl, combine cucumber, avocado, and cilantro.
9. Drizzle with olive oil and fresh lemon juice.
10. Sprinkle with salt, pepper, and cumin, then toss gently.
11. Serve chilled or at room temperature.

This salad is ideal for Pitta types, providing cooling and hydrating benefits while supporting digestion. The avocado offers healthy fats, and cumin aids in digestion.

3. **Spicy Ginger-Lemon Tea** – A simple, warming beverage to stimulate digestion and boost metabolism, particularly good for Vata and Kapha doshas.

Ingredients:

- 1 inch fresh ginger root, sliced
- Juice of 1 lemon
- 1 teaspoon honey (optional)
- 2 cups water

Method:

5. Bring water to a boil, then add ginger slices.

6. Reduce heat and simmer for 5–10 minutes.
7. Remove from heat, strain, and add lemon juice.
8. Stir in honey if desired.
9. Serve hot.

This tea is ideal for stimulating digestion and balancing Kapha's tendency toward sluggish digestion. Ginger adds warmth and zest, while lemon aids in detoxification.

In Ayurveda, the right food combinations are key to unlocking the full potential of your digestive system and achieving a balanced state of health. By aligning your food choices with your dosha and following Ayurvedic principles, you can enhance digestion, boost vitality, and support long-term well-being. Whether through comforting dishes like Kitchari, cooling salads for Pitta, or stimulating teas for Kapha, Ayurvedic recipes are designed to nourish the body, calm the mind, and restore balance.

Healing Herbs and Spices

In Ayurveda, herbs and spices are considered the cornerstone of healing. They are used not only to enhance the flavor of food but also to promote health, balance the doshas, and support the body's natural ability to heal itself. Each herb and spice has unique therapeutic properties, and they are often selected based on the specific needs of the individual, as well as the balance of the doshas. Whether in the form of teas, powders, or oils, these natural ingredients help restore harmony within the body, mind, and spirit.

Turmeric

One of the most well-known and widely used Ayurvedic herbs, **turmeric** is celebrated for its powerful anti-inflammatory and antioxidant properties. The active compound in turmeric, **curcumin**, helps reduce inflammation, detoxify the body, and improve digestion. It is often used to treat conditions like arthritis, digestive disorders, and skin ailments. Turmeric is also believed to enhance Agni (digestive fire), stimulate circulation, and support healthy liver function. It can be consumed in food, as a tea, or as a supplement to reap its benefits.

Ginger

Ginger is another staple in Ayurvedic medicine, known for its ability to stimulate digestion and balance the doshas, particularly Vata and Kapha. It is often used to treat nausea, bloating, and digestive discomfort. Ginger has a warming nature, which makes it ideal for stimulating Agni, improving circulation, and alleviating symptoms of indigestion. It also has antimicrobial properties, which help boost the immune system and fight infections. Fresh ginger can be added to teas, soups, and curries, or taken in small amounts to soothe nausea or cold-related symptoms.

Ashwagandha

Ashwagandha, also known as **Indian ginseng**, is an adaptogenic herb that helps the body adapt to stress. It is particularly useful for calming Pitta and Vata doshas. Ashwagandha is believed to support the adrenal glands, reduce anxiety, enhance mental clarity, and improve overall energy levels. It is often used as a natural remedy for stress, fatigue, and insomnia. As a grounding and rejuvenating herb, it is typically consumed in powder form, either mixed with warm milk or water, or taken as a supplement to improve stamina and vitality.

Holy Basil (Tulsi)

Tulsi, or **holy basil**, is revered in Ayurveda for its spiritual and medicinal properties.

Known as the "queen of herbs," Tulsi is highly regarded for its ability to strengthen the immune system, reduce stress, and promote mental clarity. It is often used to treat respiratory issues such as coughs, colds, and asthma, as it has anti-inflammatory and antimicrobial properties. Tulsi also helps to balance all three doshas, though it is especially beneficial for Pitta, as it has a cooling effect on the body and mind. Consuming Tulsi in the form of tea or incorporating it into food can provide a sense of calm and vitality.

Cumin
Cumin is another common spice in Ayurvedic cooking, known for its ability to stimulate digestion and enhance Agni. It is often used to treat indigestion, bloating, and gas. Cumin is warming in nature and is considered beneficial for balancing Vata dosha, which can sometimes lead to digestive disturbances. It helps promote the secretion of digestive enzymes, facilitates the absorption of nutrients, and detoxifies the liver. Cumin is frequently used in Ayurvedic formulations, teas, and soups, and it pairs well with other spices like coriander and fennel to aid digestion.

Cardamom
Cardamom, known as the "queen of spices," is a fragrant herb that has a soothing effect on the digestive system. It is especially beneficial for Pitta types, as it helps cool and calm the body and mind. Cardamom is known to promote digestion, alleviate nausea, and reduce bloating and gas. It also helps balance the mood, relieve stress, and promote mental clarity. As a digestive aid, cardamom is often added to teas, smoothies, or sweets to support overall health and soothe the digestive tract.

Coriander
Coriander is a versatile herb that is used in Ayurvedic medicine to balance all three doshas, though it is particularly effective in calming Pitta. It has cooling properties, which make it ideal for addressing conditions such as inflammation, fever, and digestive upset caused by excess heat in the body. Coriander helps improve digestion, ease nausea, and cleanse the liver. Its seeds are often ground into a powder and used in cooking or as part of Ayurvedic herbal teas.

Fennel
Fennel is a gentle, cooling herb that is particularly helpful for digestive health. It is known for its ability to reduce bloating, gas, and indigestion, making it especially beneficial for Vata and Kapha doshas. Fennel seeds can be chewed after meals to promote digestion or brewed into a tea to relieve digestive discomfort. Additionally, fennel is used to balance hormones, detoxify the body, and improve metabolism. Its mildly sweet flavor makes it a favorite in Ayurvedic cooking and teas.

Mustard Seeds
Mustard seeds are warming and stimulating, making them beneficial for Kapha and Vata

doshas. They are often used to increase circulation, clear congestion, and promote digestion. Mustard seeds are known for their ability to relieve cold symptoms and support the respiratory system. When used in cooking or as a remedy for cold-related issues, they can help promote sweating and relieve mucus buildup. Mustard oil, which is derived from the seeds, is also used in Ayurvedic massage to warm the muscles and alleviate stiffness.

Neem
Neem is considered one of the most powerful detoxifying herbs in Ayurveda. It is known for its antibacterial, antiviral, and antifungal properties. Neem is often used to cleanse the blood, purify the skin, and support liver health. It is also beneficial for balancing Pitta, as it has cooling and soothing properties. Neem can be consumed as a supplement, applied topically for skin conditions, or brewed as a tea to support overall detoxification.

Herbs and spices are an integral part of Ayurvedic medicine, offering a natural and holistic approach to healing. By incorporating these healing herbs into your diet or using them as remedies, you can support your body's natural ability to detoxify, balance the doshas, and improve digestion. From turmeric and ginger for inflammation and digestion to ashwagandha and holy basil for stress relief, these natural ingredients provide a wealth of benefits. Whether used in cooking, teas, or supplements, the therapeutic power of Ayurvedic herbs and spices helps restore harmony within the body and enhance overall well-being.

Ayurveda and Detoxification

In Ayurveda, detoxification is a vital part of maintaining health and preventing disease. The body is constantly exposed to toxins, or **Ama**, which can accumulate due to poor diet, stress, environmental factors, and emotional imbalances. Ama is believed to be the root cause of most diseases, as it disrupts the body's natural processes and hinders digestion. To restore balance and promote vitality, Ayurveda emphasizes cleansing the body through gentle, natural detoxification practices. These methods not only eliminate physical toxins but also purify the mind and spirit, helping to maintain harmony within the body.

Panchakarma: The Ayurvedic Detoxification Method
The most renowned Ayurvedic detoxification process is **Panchakarma**, a series of five therapeutic treatments designed to purify the body and rejuvenate the mind. Panchakarma involves both internal and external therapies that cleanse and balance the doshas. The process typically begins with **preparatory treatments** to loosen toxins from the tissues and prepare the body for deeper cleansing. These treatments include **abhyanga** (oil massage), **swedana** (steam therapy), and **dietary changes**.

Once the toxins have been mobilized, the main detoxification therapies are performed:

1. **Vamana (therapeutic vomiting)** – Used primarily to eliminate excess **Kapha** and clear the respiratory system. It is typically recommended for individuals with chronic congestion or digestive issues.
2. **Virechana (purgation)** – Involves the use of herbal laxatives to eliminate **Pitta** toxins from the body. It is beneficial for digestive issues, liver imbalances, or skin conditions caused by excess heat.
3. **Basti (enema therapy)** – A method of detoxifying the large intestine by introducing medicated oils or herbal decoctions. It is used to cleanse **Vata** and address conditions like constipation, bloating, or imbalances in the nervous system.
4. **Nasya (nasal administration of herbal oils)** – This treatment clears toxins from the head and sinuses and is used to address conditions like sinus congestion, headaches, and allergies.
5. **Raktamokshana (bloodletting)** – A method used to eliminate toxins from the bloodstream and is often used for skin conditions, high blood pressure, or autoimmune disorders.

Panchakarma is highly personalized, as it considers an individual's dosha, health condition, and lifestyle. The goal is to remove accumulated toxins and restore balance to the body's natural functions.

Dietary Approaches to Detoxification

In Ayurveda, food plays a crucial role in detoxification. A detoxifying diet is typically simple, light, and easy to digest, designed to support the body's natural cleansing processes. The key is to focus on **fresh, whole foods** that promote digestion, support the liver, and reduce the buildup of Ama.

- **Kitchari**: A traditional Ayurvedic dish made from rice and mung dal, Kitchari is often used in detoxification cleanses. It is light, easy to digest, and offers nourishment while allowing the body to rest and rejuvenate.
- **Herbal teas**: Detoxifying herbs like **ginger**, **turmeric**, **coriander**, and **fennel** help stimulate digestion, reduce inflammation, and support the liver. Drinking these herbal teas throughout the day aids in the elimination of toxins and improves overall digestion.
- **Warm, cooked foods**: Ayurveda emphasizes the importance of consuming warm, cooked foods during detoxification. These foods are easier to digest and help stimulate Agni, the digestive fire. Avoiding raw, cold, or processed foods is key to minimizing the burden on the digestive system.

Fasting and Food Timing

Incorporating intermittent fasting or reducing the quantity of food eaten is also part of Ayurvedic detox. Ayurveda recommends giving the digestive system a break by consuming only light, easily digestible foods, allowing the body to focus on elimination rather than digestion. It is also important to eat during the **optimal digestive hours**—lunch should be the largest meal of the day, when digestion is strongest, and dinner should be lighter and consumed early to allow for proper digestion before bedtime.

Cleansing the Mind

Detoxification in Ayurveda is not just about cleansing the body; it also involves purifying the mind and emotions. Mental and emotional toxins, such as stress, anger, or unresolved trauma, can contribute to physical imbalances and the accumulation of Ama. Ayurveda encourages practices like **meditation**, **yoga**, and **breathing exercises** (pranayama) to clear the mind and reduce mental clutter.

Herbal Support for Detoxification

Ayurvedic herbs are also frequently used to support detoxification. Herbs such as **Triphala, Turmeric, Guggulu**, and **Neem** are commonly recommended for their ability to cleanse the liver, improve digestion, and purify the blood. Triphala, a combination of three fruits—**Amla, Bibhitaki**, and **Haritaki**—is particularly popular for its gentle detoxifying effects on the digestive system, helping to eliminate waste without causing harsh purging.

- **Turmeric**: Known for its anti-inflammatory and antioxidant properties, turmeric supports liver detoxification and enhances the body's ability to eliminate toxins.
- **Neem**: Often used for skin conditions and detoxification, Neem purifies the blood and supports the immune system.
- **Guggulu**: This resin is commonly used to detoxify the lymphatic system and promote healthy circulation.

Practical Detox Tips in Ayurveda
To support detoxification in daily life, Ayurveda offers several practical tips:

1. **Start the day with warm water**: Drinking warm water with lemon or ginger helps stimulate digestion and cleanse the body.
2. **Practice oil pulling**: Swishing oil (usually sesame or coconut oil) in the mouth for several minutes can help remove toxins from the oral cavity and improve oral hygiene.
3. **Self-massage (Abhyanga)**: Daily self-massage with warm oil improves circulation, helps eliminate toxins, and promotes relaxation.
4. **Get adequate rest**: Sleep is essential for detoxification, as the body repairs and cleanses itself during rest.

In Ayurveda, detoxification is viewed as a holistic process that involves not only cleansing the body of toxins but also nourishing the mind and spirit. Through personalized methods like Panchakarma, dietary adjustments, herbal support, and mental clarity practices, Ayurveda provides a comprehensive approach to purifying the body and restoring balance. By incorporating these practices into daily life, individuals can improve digestion, enhance vitality, and support long-term health, creating a natural path to healing and rejuvenation.

Purification Procedures in Ayurveda

In Ayurveda, purification is a central concept for maintaining health, as it aims to eliminate accumulated toxins (Ama) that can obstruct the body's natural flow and lead to illness. The purification procedures in Ayurveda are designed to cleanse not just the body, but also the mind and spirit, fostering overall well-being and balance. These procedures focus on restoring harmony between the body's internal environment and the external world, ensuring optimal function of the digestive system, immunity, and metabolism. Among the many purification techniques in Ayurveda, **Panchakarma** is the most well-known, but there are other supportive practices that play a vital role in detoxifying and rejuvenating the body.

Panchakarma: The Fivefold Detoxification

Panchakarma, meaning "five actions," is the primary Ayurvedic detoxification and rejuvenation procedure. It involves a series of therapeutic treatments that help eliminate toxins, promote healing, and restore balance to the body. The process typically includes three main stages: **preparatory treatments**, the **main therapies**, and **post-treatment rejuvenation**.

1. **Preparatory Treatments**
   Before the main detoxification procedures, the body must be prepared to release toxins. This phase involves two key practices:
   - **Snehana (oleation)**: The body is massaged with warm medicated oils to loosen and lubricate the tissues, soften accumulated toxins, and prepare the digestive system for deeper cleansing. This treatment helps calm the nervous system and promotes relaxation.
   - **Swedana (sudation)**: After oleation, the body is exposed to steam or heat therapy to open the pores, increase perspiration, and further loosen toxins. The combination of oil and steam helps to deeply penetrate the tissues, making it easier to eliminate waste.
2. **The Main Panchakarma Therapies**
   Once the body is prepared, the main cleansing therapies are performed, tailored to the individual's doshic constitution and current imbalances.
   - **Vamana (therapeutic vomiting)**: This procedure is used to eliminate excess **Kapha** and clear the respiratory tract. Vamana is particularly helpful for individuals suffering from respiratory issues, chronic cough, asthma, or excess mucus in the body.

- **Virechana (purgation)**: This treatment involves the use of purgative herbs to eliminate **Pitta** from the body, particularly from the liver and gallbladder. It is commonly used to treat digestive issues, skin conditions, and conditions caused by excess heat or inflammation, such as acne or ulcers.
- **Basti (enema therapy)**: Used to cleanse the colon and restore balance to **Vata**, Basti is one of the most important therapies in Panchakarma. It is done with herbal oils, decoctions, or other medicinal liquids that are introduced into the rectum to cleanse the digestive system, lubricate the tissues, and strengthen the body's elimination processes. It is especially beneficial for constipation, gas, bloating, and inflammatory bowel disorders.
- **Nasya (nasal therapy)**: Nasya involves the administration of medicated oils or powders through the nose to cleanse the sinuses, head, and neck. This procedure is useful for addressing sinus congestion, headaches, migraines, allergies, and mental clarity issues. Nasya is thought to balance **Kapha** in the head and improve overall mental function.
- **Raktamokshana (bloodletting)**: A more specialized therapy used to purify the blood, Raktamokshana helps eliminate toxins that have been accumulated in the bloodstream. It is typically used for skin conditions, certain types of fever, and to treat conditions related to excess blood or toxicity.

3. **Post-Treatment Rejuvenation**
After the detoxification process, it is crucial to restore balance and rejuvenate the body. This phase includes gentle therapies that help rebuild strength, improve digestion, and prevent further imbalances.
    - **Abhyanga (oil massage)**: A soothing oil massage with herbs can help relax the body, promote circulation, and maintain the effects of detoxification. Abhyanga is often done with warm medicated oils to nourish and hydrate the skin while soothing the nervous system.
    - **Rasayana (rejuvenation therapy)**: Following Panchakarma, Rasayana therapies focus on restoring the body's vitality and improving overall health. This includes the use of rejuvenating herbs like **Ashwagandha** and **Amalaki**, which support immunity, enhance energy levels, and promote longevity.

Diet and Lifestyle Adjustments During Purification

In addition to the physical therapies, Ayurveda emphasizes the importance of diet and lifestyle changes during the purification process. During Panchakarma and other cleansing treatments, individuals are typically advised to follow a **light, easy-to-digest diet** consisting of foods that are warm, moist, and nourishing to support the body's healing process. **Kitchari**, a traditional Ayurvedic dish made from rice and mung dal, is often recommended during detoxification due to its gentle and cleansing nature.

Ayurveda also stresses the importance of adequate rest, stress management, and mindfulness during detoxification. The practice of **yoga** and **meditation** is encouraged to help cleanse the mind, reduce emotional toxins, and support the body's physical detoxification.

Other Ayurvedic Purification Techniques

Beyond Panchakarma, Ayurveda offers other purification procedures that can be incorporated into daily or seasonal routines. These practices help maintain the body's natural balance and prevent the accumulation of toxins:

- **Tongue scraping**: A daily Ayurvedic practice that removes accumulated toxins and bacteria from the surface of the tongue, improving oral health and digestion.
- **Oil pulling**: Swishing oil, typically sesame or coconut, in the mouth for several minutes to draw out toxins, improve dental health, and strengthen the immune system.
- **Self-massage (Abhyanga)**: Regular self-massage with warm oil helps stimulate circulation, promote relaxation, and maintain the balance of the doshas.

Purification procedures in Ayurveda, particularly Panchakarma, are a profound way to restore balance, detoxify the body, and rejuvenate the mind and spirit. These therapies are designed to remove toxins, optimize digestion, and promote vitality, allowing the body to heal and function at its best. By following the guidance of Ayurvedic practitioners and integrating these cleansing practices into daily life, individuals can support their body's natural detoxification processes and achieve a healthier, more balanced existence.

Importance of Detoxification

In Ayurveda, detoxification is seen as a crucial practice for maintaining health, vitality, and overall well-being. The concept of detoxification, or **Shodhana**, is based on the belief that the body is constantly exposed to toxins, or **Ama**, which can accumulate and create blockages within the digestive system, tissues, and even the mind. These toxins are considered the root cause of many diseases and imbalances, leading to conditions such as fatigue, digestive issues, skin disorders, and emotional disturbances. Therefore, regular detoxification is not only important for addressing existing health concerns but also for preventing the buildup of toxins that could lead to future health problems.

Restoring Agni: The Digestive Fire
In Ayurveda, the strength of **Agni**, or digestive fire, is central to health. Agni is responsible for transforming food into energy, absorbing nutrients, and eliminating waste. A strong Agni is necessary for proper digestion and the efficient removal of toxins from the body. However, when Agni is weak—often due to poor dietary habits, stress, or environmental factors—the body's ability to digest food properly diminishes. This leads to the accumulation of undigested food particles, or **Ama**, which can fester in the tissues and disrupt bodily functions. Detoxification helps to restore the balance of Agni, reviving the body's ability to properly digest food, absorb nutrients, and eliminate waste effectively.

Clearing Ama and Balancing the Doshas
Toxins accumulate due to a combination of poor diet, sedentary lifestyle, emotional stress, and environmental pollutants. These toxins can manifest as **Ama**, which disrupt the balance of the body's three primary energies, or **doshas**: **Vata**, **Pitta**, and **Kapha**. When these doshas become imbalanced, they can contribute to various ailments. For example:

- **Vata imbalance** often leads to dryness, constipation, and anxiety.
- **Pitta imbalance** results in inflammation, acidity, and skin conditions.
- **Kapha imbalance** can cause sluggish digestion, weight gain, and respiratory issues.

Detoxification helps clear Ama from the body and brings the doshas back into harmony. By eliminating toxins, the body is able to regain its natural equilibrium, which enhances overall health and vitality.

Enhancing Immunity and Promoting Longevity

Regular detoxification supports the body's immune system by helping it eliminate harmful substances and pollutants. When the body is free of toxins, it is better equipped to fight infections, reduce inflammation, and prevent disease. Ayurvedic detoxification practices, such as **Panchakarma, herbal cleansing**, and **dietary adjustments**, encourage the body to expel toxins, strengthen the digestive system, and promote healthy cellular regeneration. This process not only supports the immune system but also contributes to longevity by ensuring that the body remains clear of harmful substances that could otherwise shorten lifespan or lead to chronic health problems.

Improved Digestion and Better Absorption of Nutrients

A major benefit of detoxification is its ability to enhance digestion. When Ama is present in the body, it creates blockages in the digestive system, making it harder for the body to absorb nutrients effectively. Detoxification helps eliminate these blockages, allowing the digestive system to function optimally. Once toxins are cleared, the body can more efficiently absorb essential nutrients from food, leading to improved energy levels, better skin health, and overall vitality. Moreover, cleansing the digestive system also helps reduce symptoms of indigestion, bloating, and constipation, which are common signs of toxin accumulation.

Mental and Emotional Cleansing

In Ayurveda, detoxification is not limited to the physical body; it also extends to mental and emotional health. Just as the body accumulates physical toxins, the mind can accumulate emotional toxins, such as stress, anger, fear, or unresolved trauma. These emotional blockages can negatively affect one's mood, mental clarity, and overall mental health. Detoxification helps to clear these emotional blockages by promoting relaxation, reducing stress, and restoring emotional balance. Practices like **meditation**, **yoga**, and **mindful breathing** are often incorporated into Ayurvedic detox programs to support mental and emotional healing.

Panchakarma: A Comprehensive Detox Approach

One of the most effective Ayurvedic detoxification methods is **Panchakarma**, a five-fold therapy that includes a combination of body treatments, herbal remedies, and dietary changes. Panchakarma works to clear toxins from the body, restore balance to the doshas, and rejuvenate the body and mind. The therapies involved in Panchakarma are tailored to the individual's doshic constitution and health needs, ensuring a personalized and holistic approach to detoxification.

The process involves **oleation** (massaging the body with medicated oils), **steam therapy**, **purgation** (using herbs to cleanse the body), **enema therapy**, and **nasal therapy**. These therapies work synergistically to detoxify the body at both the physical and emotional levels, promoting deep healing and rejuvenation.

Supportive Detox Practices
In addition to Panchakarma, Ayurveda recommends various daily practices to maintain detoxification. These include **tongue scraping**, which removes toxins from the mouth, **oil pulling** to cleanse the oral cavity and improve dental health, and **self-massage** (Abhyanga) with warm oils to stimulate circulation and eliminate toxins through the skin. Herbal teas, such as those made with **ginger**, **turmeric**, or **Triphala**, can be consumed to aid digestion and enhance detoxification.

Detoxification is an essential practice in Ayurveda, not just for treating illness, but for preventing disease and promoting overall health. By removing toxins and improving digestion, Ayurveda ensures that the body functions at its highest potential. Regular detoxification, when practiced mindfully and in harmony with the body's needs, supports not only physical health but also emotional well-being, mental clarity, and longevity. Whether through Panchakarma, herbal remedies, or dietary adjustments, Ayurvedic detoxification helps restore balance, boost vitality, and enhance the body's natural healing capacity.

Ayurvedic Home Remedies for Detox

Ayurvedic home remedies offer simple, natural ways to detoxify the body, restore balance, and improve overall health. By harnessing the power of herbs, spices, and lifestyle practices, Ayurveda provides accessible solutions to support the body's natural detoxification processes. These remedies not only help cleanse the body of accumulated toxins (Ama) but also promote optimal digestion, boost energy levels, and enhance mental clarity. Many Ayurvedic detox practices can be easily incorporated into daily routines, allowing individuals to enjoy the benefits of detoxification from the comfort of their own homes.

Warm Water with Lemon

One of the easiest and most effective detox remedies is drinking warm water with fresh lemon juice first thing in the morning. The acidity of lemon helps stimulate the digestive system, promoting the production of digestive enzymes. Lemon is also rich in vitamin C, which aids in detoxifying the liver and enhancing its ability to process toxins. Drinking warm lemon water flushes out accumulated Ama, supports hydration, and helps restore the balance of the doshas, especially **Pitta**, which tends to become overheated. This simple habit sets a positive tone for the day by kickstarting the body's cleansing process.

Triphala

Triphala, a powerful herbal blend made from three fruits—**Amla** (Indian gooseberry), **Bibhitaki**, and **Haritaki**—is one of the most widely used Ayurvedic remedies for detoxification. Triphala is known for its ability to gently cleanse the digestive tract, promote regular bowel movements, and improve overall digestion. It works by stimulating the digestive fire (Agni), removing waste products from the colon, and clearing toxins from the body. Triphala can be taken in powdered or tablet form, typically before bed, to encourage effective elimination overnight. It is considered a safe, non-habit-forming remedy for detoxification and general digestive health.

Ginger and Turmeric Tea

A blend of **ginger** and **turmeric** makes an excellent detoxifying tea, especially for those dealing with inflammation, digestive issues, or sluggish metabolism. Ginger is known for its ability to stimulate digestion, reduce bloating, and clear accumulated toxins, while turmeric is a powerful anti-inflammatory herb that supports liver function and promotes detoxification. To make the tea, simply steep fresh ginger slices and a pinch of turmeric in hot water, and add a little honey or lemon for taste. This warming tea is especially beneficial for **Vata** and **Pitta** types, as it helps balance their digestive systems and clears excess heat or dryness.

Coriander, Cumin, and Fennel Tea

This traditional Ayurvedic herbal tea blend is often recommended to aid digestion, reduce bloating, and improve detoxification. **Coriander** helps to balance the **Pitta** dosha by cooling the body, while **cumin** and **fennel** stimulate the digestive fire (Agni), helping to break down food more efficiently. These herbs are known to support healthy digestion, enhance nutrient absorption, and prevent the buildup of toxins in the body. To make the tea, combine equal parts of ground cumin, coriander, and fennel seeds, steep in hot water, and sip throughout the day for a gentle detox.

Apple Cider Vinegar

Apple cider vinegar is a popular remedy in Ayurveda for stimulating digestion, alkalizing the body, and promoting detoxification. It is believed to help balance the **Kapha** dosha, particularly in cases of excess mucus or sluggish digestion. The acetic acid in apple cider vinegar aids in breaking down food, promoting better absorption of nutrients, and flushing out toxins. To use, dilute 1–2 tablespoons of apple cider vinegar in a glass of warm water and drink it before meals to improve digestion and support the liver's detoxifying functions.

Castor Oil for Bowel Health

Castor oil is a potent Ayurvedic remedy used to clear toxins from the digestive system. It is particularly effective in detoxifying the colon and improving the elimination of waste. Castor oil has a mild laxative effect and is typically used for a **Vata** or **Kapha** imbalance. It helps relieve constipation, promotes the removal of accumulated Ama, and supports liver detoxification. To use, take 1–2 teaspoons of cold-pressed castor oil before bedtime, but be cautious as it can have a strong purging effect. This remedy is best used occasionally or under the guidance of an Ayurvedic practitioner.

Pineapple and Mint Smoothie

Pineapple contains **bromelain**, an enzyme that helps break down proteins and promotes efficient digestion. Paired with **mint**, which has a cooling effect on the digestive system and helps reduce inflammation, this smoothie serves as a gentle digestive aid and a tasty detox treat. Pineapple and mint are especially useful for **Pitta** types, as they help clear heat and support the liver's detoxification process. To make the smoothie, blend fresh pineapple, mint leaves, and a little coconut water for a refreshing, detoxifying drink that can be enjoyed as a snack or light breakfast.

Self-Massage (Abhyanga) with Herbal Oils

Abhyanga, or self-massage with warm herbal oils, is a highly effective Ayurvedic practice for promoting circulation, reducing stress, and aiding detoxification. The process involves massaging the body with warm oil infused with herbs like **turmeric**, **ginger**, or

neem to stimulate the lymphatic system, eliminate toxins, and nourish the skin. Regular self-massage improves blood flow, reduces muscle stiffness, and enhances the body's ability to eliminate waste. It is particularly beneficial for **Vata** types, who often experience dryness and stiffness, and for **Kapha** types, who may benefit from improved circulation and energy flow.

Fasting or Intermittent Fasting

Fasting is another powerful detox tool in Ayurveda, especially when done mindfully and under proper guidance. Ayurveda recommends fasting as a way to allow the body's digestive system to rest, repair, and eliminate toxins. One of the most common fasting practices is **intermittent fasting**, where meals are consumed during a specific window of time, allowing the body to focus on detoxification outside of eating hours. Fasting encourages the body to burn stored toxins, and it is often combined with herbal teas or light, easy-to-digest foods to support the detox process. However, it is important to approach fasting carefully, especially for those with underlying health conditions.

Ayurvedic home remedies for detoxification offer natural, holistic methods for purging toxins from the body, improving digestion, and restoring balance to the doshas. By incorporating simple practices like drinking herbal teas, using detoxifying foods and herbs, and engaging in self-care routines such as Abhyanga, individuals can support their body's natural detox processes without the need for harsh chemicals or invasive procedures. Ayurveda's approach to detox is gentle, personalized, and sustainable, making it a valuable tool for long-term health and wellness.

Ayurveda and Yoga

Ayurveda and yoga are two ancient systems of wellness that are deeply intertwined, each complementing the other to foster physical, mental, and spiritual health. Both traditions originate from the same Vedic texts and share a common goal: to achieve balance and harmony within the body and mind. While Ayurveda focuses on the physical and medicinal aspects of health, yoga offers tools for mental clarity, flexibility, and spiritual growth. Together, they form a holistic approach to well-being that integrates body, mind, and spirit, allowing individuals to lead a life of vitality, peace, and inner harmony.

In Ayurveda, health is seen as the balance between the body's internal energies or **doshas**: Vata, Pitta, and Kapha. Each dosha represents different elements and functions within the body and mind. When these energies are in balance, a person experiences good health, but when they are imbalanced, disease can occur. Similarly, in yoga, the emphasis is placed on the balance of energies, particularly through the regulation of **prana** (life force energy), breath control (pranayama), and the practice of asanas (physical postures). Yoga helps balance the doshas by promoting the free flow of prana throughout the body, thus enhancing physical health and mental clarity.

The Role of Yoga in Balancing the Doshas

Yoga practice is personalized according to an individual's doshic constitution. Different postures, breathing exercises, and meditative techniques can be tailored to address the unique needs of each dosha, helping to maintain equilibrium and prevent imbalances.

- **Vata**: Vata types, characterized by qualities of dryness, coldness, and lightness, often need grounding and stabilizing practices. Gentle and restorative yoga poses that promote relaxation and calm the nervous system are beneficial for Vata individuals. **Standing poses, seated forward bends**, and **prone postures** that provide stability and warmth help balance Vata. Pranayama practices like **Nadi Shodhana** (alternate nostril breathing) are also effective in calming the nervous system and calming an overactive mind.
- **Pitta**: Pitta types, who are fiery and intense, require cooling, calming, and soothing yoga practices. Poses that reduce heat and promote relaxation are ideal for balancing Pitta, such as **forward bends, hip openers**, and **restorative poses** like **child's pose**. Pranayama techniques such as **Ujjayi breath** (victorious breath) and **Sitali breath** (cooling breath) are effective for cooling Pitta's internal heat

and reducing stress. Pitta types should also avoid overly intense or competitive practices that can trigger excess fire.
- **Kapha**: Kapha types, known for their stability and tendency to accumulate weight, benefit from dynamic, invigorating yoga practices that stimulate circulation and reduce sluggishness. **Vinyasa** or **flow-based practices**, including **sun salutations**, are great for Kapha types as they engage the body in movement, helping to balance the heaviness and increase energy levels. Standing poses, **backbends**, and **twists** also help to open up the body and release stored tension. **Kapalbhati** (skull-shining breath) is a powerful pranayama technique to invigorate Kapha, clear congestion, and stimulate the digestive fire.

Pranayama: Breath Control for Energy Balance

Breathing exercises, or **pranayama**, play an essential role in both Ayurveda and yoga by controlling the flow of prana (life force energy) within the body. The breath is seen as the link between the body and the mind, and by regulating the breath, an individual can influence their physical and mental state.

- For **Vata** individuals, pranayama practices should focus on calming and grounding the breath. Techniques like **Nadi Shodhana** (alternate nostril breathing) or **Bhramari** (bee breath) are ideal, as they calm the nervous system and help settle an overactive mind.
- For **Pitta**, cooling breaths such as **Sitali** (cooling breath) or **Ujjayi** (victorious breath) are excellent for reducing internal heat and calming an agitated mind.
- For **Kapha**, stimulating techniques such as **Kapalbhati** (skull-shining breath) and **Bhastrika** (bellows breath) help clear congestion, boost metabolism, and increase energy levels.

Ayurveda's Influence on Yoga Practice

Ayurveda provides important insights into how to approach yoga with an awareness of the body's constitution and imbalances. Ayurvedic principles influence the way yoga is practiced by encouraging the selection of the right time, environment, and type of practice suited to an individual's constitution and lifestyle.

- **Timing**: According to Ayurveda, the best time for practicing yoga is during the **Kapha time** of day (from 6 AM to 10 AM), when the energy is steady and calm. Yoga in the morning helps activate the body and mind, promoting circulation and mental clarity.
- **Diet and Nutrition**: Ayurveda emphasizes that a balanced diet supports yoga practice. For instance, Vata types should eat warm, moist, and grounding foods to balance their tendency toward dryness, while Pitta types should consume cooling foods to balance their fiery nature. Kapha individuals are advised to eat lighter, stimulating foods that support their metabolism. Ayurveda also suggests that the

practice of yoga should be followed by appropriate nutrition to support the body's energy needs and recovery.
- **Postures**: Different yoga asanas (postures) are also recommended based on an individual's dosha. For example, **restorative poses** such as **supta baddha konasana** (reclining bound angle pose) help Vata types relax and feel grounded, while **dynamic sequences** like **sun salutations** can help Kapha types get energized.

Meditation: The Mental Detox

Yoga and meditation are integral components of Ayurveda's approach to mental and emotional well-being. Meditation helps clear mental toxins, reduce stress, and cultivate a peaceful mind. **Mindfulness meditation** and **mantra meditation** are commonly used to calm the mind, enhance clarity, and promote emotional balance. By integrating yoga with meditation, an individual can achieve a holistic balance of body, mind, and spirit.

Ayurveda suggests that mental toxins, such as stress, anxiety, and fear, can contribute to physical imbalances in the body. Meditation works to alleviate these emotional toxins, creating mental space for healing and balance.

The synergy between Ayurveda and yoga provides a comprehensive approach to health, offering tools that nurture the body, mind, and spirit. While Ayurveda provides the knowledge of how to balance the doshas through diet, herbs, and lifestyle, yoga offers the physical and mental practices that support that balance. Together, they create a powerful system for holistic wellness, addressing not only the physical body but also emotional and spiritual aspects of health. By practicing yoga with an awareness of one's Ayurvedic constitution, individuals can promote overall well-being, cultivate balance, and achieve lasting harmony in their lives.

Yoga Postures for Your Dosha

In Ayurveda, each individual has a unique constitution, or **Prakriti**, determined by the balance of the three doshas: **Vata**, **Pitta**, and **Kapha**. These doshas influence not only physical traits but also mental and emotional tendencies. Yoga, with its physical postures (asanas), breathing exercises (pranayama), and meditation, is a powerful tool in Ayurveda for balancing the doshas and promoting overall health. Specific yoga postures are recommended based on an individual's doshic constitution to help bring the body into harmony, improve digestion, and reduce stress.

Yoga for Vata

Vata is characterized by qualities of dryness, lightness, and coldness. People with a dominant Vata dosha tend to be energetic, creative, and quick-witted, but they may also experience anxiety, restlessness, and dryness in the body, particularly in the joints and skin. Vata types benefit from grounding, warming, and stabilizing practices in yoga that calm the nervous system, improve circulation, and promote relaxation.

- **Seated Forward Bend (Paschimottanasana)**: This forward fold stretches the hamstrings, calms the nervous system, and helps to ground Vata types. The forward bending action can also help release tension and promote relaxation.
- **Tree Pose (Vrksasana)**: As a balancing posture, Tree Pose helps stabilize Vata, promoting mental and physical grounding. It improves focus and concentration, which is essential for Vata's often scattered energy.
- **Child's Pose (Balasana)**: A restorative pose, Child's Pose is excellent for Vata types who need to calm down and release stress. The forward fold and gentle stretching help soothe the nervous system, ease lower back tension, and improve mental clarity.
- **Legs Up the Wall Pose (Viparita Karani)**: This pose promotes relaxation and stability, relieving tension and calming the mind. It's particularly useful for Vata types who tend to have restless energy or experience anxiety.

Yoga for Pitta

Pitta is the dosha associated with heat, intensity, and transformation. Pitta types are driven, focused, and energetic but can become easily irritated, overheated, and stressed. Yoga postures for Pitta should be cooling, calming, and designed to release excess heat from the body and mind while reducing stress and inflammation.

- **Cobra Pose (Bhujangasana)**: This backbend opens the chest and stimulates the digestive system while releasing tension in the upper body. It is a cooling posture that encourages an expansive, open feeling, counteracting Pitta's tendency toward tightness and excess heat.
- **Child's Pose (Balasana)**: Again, this pose is beneficial for Pitta to relieve mental and physical stress. It cools the body and calms the mind, helping Pitta types manage their fiery energy.
- **Downward-Facing Dog (Adho Mukha Svanasana)**: A cooling inversion that releases tension from the upper body while strengthening and stretching the legs. This pose helps bring balance to Pitta by offering a release for accumulated tension, particularly around the shoulders and neck.
- **Seated Spinal Twist (Ardha Matsyendrasana)**: Twists help improve digestion, promote detoxification, and relieve tension from the spine. This pose encourages release and relaxation, both physically and mentally, reducing excess heat and stress.

Yoga for Kapha

Kapha is associated with stability, structure, and calmness but can become sluggish, lethargic, and prone to weight gain when out of balance. Kapha types often need energizing and stimulating yoga practices that encourage movement, flexibility, and metabolic stimulation to overcome the heavy, slow qualities of this dosha.

- **Sun Salutations (Surya Namaskar)**: A dynamic sequence of poses that warms the body and gets the heart rate up. This series is energizing and stimulates circulation, helping to break up Kapha's tendency toward stagnation and sluggishness.
- **Warrior Poses (Virabhadrasana I & II)**: These standing poses help build strength, stamina, and energy. The action of lunging forward in Warrior Pose is perfect for Kapha, helping to open the hips, stimulate the legs, and energize the entire body.
- **Bridge Pose (Setu Bandhasana)**: This backbend opens the chest and lungs while stimulating the thyroid and energizing the body. It helps Kapha release heaviness, particularly around the chest and diaphragm, and provides a sense of lightness and vitality.
- **Standing Forward Bend (Uttanasana)**: This pose stretches the hamstrings and lengthens the spine while calming the nervous system. It also promotes blood circulation and helps relieve mental and physical tension, which is especially beneficial for Kapha types who may feel sluggish or stuck.

Pranayama for Dosha Balance

Breathing exercises, or **pranayama**, play an important role in balancing the doshas through the regulation of prana (life force energy). Each dosha benefits from specific breathwork techniques that support its qualities and restore balance.

- **Vata**: For Vata, **Nadi Shodhana** (alternate nostril breathing) is particularly helpful as it calms the nervous system, reduces anxiety, and helps focus scattered energy. **Bhramari** (bee breath) is another beneficial technique for calming the mind and promoting relaxation.
- **Pitta**: **Ujjayi breath** (victorious breath) can help Pitta types by soothing excess heat and calming the mind, while **Sitali** (cooling breath) is perfect for cooling down fiery Pitta energy and reducing stress.
- **Kapha**: **Kapalbhati** (skull-shining breath) is ideal for Kapha types, as it invigorates the body, clears congestion, and stimulates the digestive system. **Bhastrika** (bellows breath) is also a great choice for stimulating energy and improving mental clarity.

Yoga postures tailored to your dosha can significantly improve your health and well-being by addressing the unique imbalances of your body and mind. By practicing specific poses that align with your doshic qualities, you can bring stability to Vata, calm Pitta, or energize Kapha. Integrating yoga with Ayurvedic principles allows you to create a holistic wellness routine that balances your physical, mental, and emotional states, helping you feel centered, healthy, and revitalized. Whether through grounding poses for Vata, cooling poses for Pitta, or energizing movements for Kapha, yoga offers the tools to enhance your Ayurveda-based lifestyle.

Ayurveda and Pranayama

In Ayurveda, breath is considered the bridge between the body and mind, and **pranayama** (breathing exercises) plays a crucial role in maintaining balance and harmony within the body's energy systems. Prana, the vital life force or energy that flows through the body, is directly influenced by the breath. Through the practice of pranayama, individuals can control the flow of prana, improving mental clarity, emotional well-being, and physical health. In Ayurveda, pranayama is used to regulate the doshas (Vata, Pitta, and Kapha) by either calming, stimulating, or balancing the energies within the body.

The Role of Breath in Ayurveda

Breath, or **Prana**, is considered essential to life in Ayurveda. The breath is not just a physical process; it is believed to be the vehicle for prana, which circulates through the body's **nadis** (energy channels) and chakras (energy centers). Pranayama, meaning "control of prana," is the practice of conscious breathing that helps enhance the flow of prana, clear energy blockages, and restore balance to the body and mind. Proper breathing helps harmonize the doshas, especially when they are imbalanced due to stress, poor lifestyle, or improper diet.

Pranayama and the Doshas

Each dosha has its own unique characteristics, and pranayama can be used to calm, stimulate, or balance the energies of the doshas. Depending on the individual's constitution or current imbalance, specific breathing techniques are recommended.

- **Vata**: Vata is associated with the qualities of dryness, coldness, and lightness. When Vata is out of balance, it can lead to symptoms like anxiety, restlessness, dryness, and digestive issues. Pranayama techniques for Vata focus on grounding, calming, and nourishing the nervous system to reduce excessive movement and erratic energy.
    - **Nadi Shodhana** (Alternate Nostril Breathing): This technique is particularly beneficial for Vata, as it calms the nervous system, reduces stress, and helps balance the mind and emotions.
    - **Bhramari** (Bee Breath): This calming pranayama technique involves producing a humming sound while exhaling. It helps soothe the mind,

- relieve anxiety, and promote mental clarity, making it ideal for Vata types who may experience overactive thoughts and worry.
- **Pitta**: Pitta is linked with heat, intensity, and transformation. When Pitta is aggravated, it can lead to conditions such as irritability, inflammation, acidity, and skin issues. Pranayama for Pitta focuses on cooling, soothing, and calming the fiery energy within the body.
    - **Ujjayi Breath** (Victorious Breath): This technique is effective for calming Pitta by generating a soothing, cooling sensation within the body. It helps regulate the flow of energy and promotes focus, making it ideal for those who feel overheated or overly driven.
    - **Sitali Breath** (Cooling Breath): Sitali is a cooling pranayama technique that involves inhaling through the mouth and exhaling through the nose. This breath helps to cool the body, calm the mind, and reduce excess heat, making it particularly beneficial for Pitta imbalances.
- **Kapha**: Kapha is associated with stability, heaviness, and sluggishness. When Kapha becomes imbalanced, it can lead to lethargy, weight gain, and congestion. Pranayama for Kapha focuses on stimulating, energizing, and clearing blockages to boost circulation and reduce excess heaviness.
    - **Kapalbhati** (Skull-Shining Breath): This invigorating technique involves forceful exhalations followed by passive inhalations. Kapalbhati stimulates the digestive fire (Agni), clears the sinuses, and promotes mental clarity. It is perfect for Kapha types, as it increases energy and helps alleviate sluggishness.
    - **Bhastrika** (Bellows Breath): This technique involves rapid, forceful inhalations and exhalations, which helps to stimulate the body, increase heat, and reduce congestion. Bhastrika energizes Kapha, clearing out stagnant energy and improving focus.

The Benefits of Pranayama in Ayurveda

Pranayama has a range of therapeutic benefits, both physical and mental, that align with Ayurvedic principles of health. The practice of conscious breathing enhances **Agni** (digestive fire), reduces **Ama** (toxins), and helps balance the doshas.

- **Improved Digestion**: By stimulating the parasympathetic nervous system, pranayama helps to improve digestion and enhance the body's ability to absorb nutrients. Certain breathing techniques, such as **Kapalbhati**, are particularly useful for increasing Agni and promoting healthy digestion.
- **Stress Reduction**: Ayurveda views stress as one of the primary causes of disease, particularly when it disturbs the natural flow of prana and leads to dosha imbalances. Pranayama calms the mind and body, reducing cortisol levels, anxiety, and mental fatigue, which helps maintain emotional balance.

- **Enhanced Circulation**: Pranayama improves blood circulation and oxygenates the body's tissues, providing more energy and vitality. Techniques like **Nadi Shodhana** can also help balance the flow of energy through the body's nadis, ensuring that prana moves freely and harmoniously.
- **Mental Clarity and Focus**: Pranayama clears mental fog, sharpens concentration, and enhances memory. For Pitta types, breathing exercises like **Ujjayi** and **Bhramari** help calm an overactive mind, while for Vata, they help reduce the tendency for mental restlessness.

The Integration of Pranayama with Ayurvedic Practices

In Ayurveda, lifestyle and dietary choices are just as important as breathwork when it comes to balancing the doshas and promoting overall health. Pranayama can be combined with other Ayurvedic practices, such as:

- **Diet**: Eating foods that align with your dosha helps maintain the body's internal balance. For instance, Vata types should eat warm, moist foods, while Pitta types benefit from cooling foods and Kapha types should focus on light and stimulating meals. Combining a balanced diet with pranayama enhances digestion and detoxification.
- **Herbal Remedies**: Many Ayurvedic herbs like **Ashwagandha**, **Triphala**, and **Tulsi** can support the effects of pranayama, calming the mind and boosting energy. Herbal teas can be consumed before or after pranayama practice to promote detoxification and relaxation.
- **Meditation and Yoga**: Both Ayurveda and yoga share a common foundation in promoting harmony of the body, mind, and spirit. Incorporating pranayama into a regular yoga practice and combining it with meditation can deepen the detoxifying effects and bring about greater emotional balance and mental clarity.

Pranayama in Ayurveda is more than just a breathing exercise; it is a vital tool for maintaining the flow of prana throughout the body, balancing the doshas, and supporting physical and mental health. Whether you are looking to calm an overactive mind, improve digestion, or increase energy, pranayama offers a variety of techniques to suit your unique constitution. By integrating pranayama into your daily routine, alongside Ayurvedic lifestyle practices, you can restore balance, improve vitality, and achieve lasting wellness.

Meditation Techniques in Ayurveda

In Ayurveda, meditation is considered an essential practice for mental clarity, emotional stability, and overall health. The mind, much like the body, is believed to be affected by imbalances, which can manifest as stress, anxiety, or confusion. Ayurveda sees meditation as a powerful tool to calm the mind, reduce these imbalances, and promote the smooth flow of **prana** (life force energy) throughout the body. Various meditation techniques are recommended based on an individual's doshic constitution, with the goal of bringing harmony to both mind and body.

Meditation for Vata

Vata types are characterized by qualities of lightness, dryness, and restlessness. Their minds can often become scattered, leading to anxiety, overthinking, and difficulty focusing. To balance Vata, meditation practices should focus on grounding, centering, and calming the nervous system.

- **Visualization Meditation**: For Vata, guided visualization is an excellent technique. This involves imagining calming, stable images such as a tree with deep roots or a peaceful, quiet landscape. Visualization helps to calm the restless mind and anchor it in the present moment, promoting mental stability.
- **Mantra Meditation**: Repeating a mantra like **"So Hum"** (I am that) or a simple sound can help Vata types find focus and reduce mental agitation. The rhythmic repetition of sound has a calming effect and helps to settle the busy mind, creating a sense of grounding.
- **Breathing Techniques**: **Nadi Shodhana** (alternate nostril breathing) is particularly effective for Vata, as it calms the nervous system, clears mental fog, and promotes balance. This practice helps to regulate the flow of prana and enhances mental clarity, which is beneficial for Vata types who may struggle with scattered thoughts.

Meditation for Pitta

Pitta is associated with heat, intensity, and focus. Pitta types are often driven, intelligent, and goal-oriented, but they can become overheated, irritable, or aggressive when out of balance. The goal of meditation for Pitta is to cool the mind, reduce stress, and foster relaxation.

- **Breathing Techniques**: **Sitali** (cooling breath) and **Ujjayi** (victorious breath) are beneficial for Pitta types. Sitali involves inhaling through the mouth, which creates a cooling effect on the body and mind. Ujjayi breath helps reduce stress and provides a calming focus. These breathing techniques help Pitta types manage their internal heat and keep their minds calm.
- **Silent Meditation**: Silent sitting or mindfulness meditation is an excellent way for Pitta types to cultivate inner peace. The practice involves focusing on the breath and letting thoughts come and go without attachment. This practice helps Pitta types move away from their driven, goal-oriented nature and tap into stillness and peace.
- **Loving Kindness Meditation (Metta)**: This technique, also known as **Metta Bhavana**, involves focusing on sending feelings of love, compassion, and kindness to oneself and others. For Pitta types, who can sometimes struggle with perfectionism or frustration, this practice fosters patience, reduces anger, and promotes emotional balance.

Meditation for Kapha

Kapha is characterized by qualities of heaviness, stability, and calmness. Kapha types tend to be grounded and patient, but when imbalanced, they can become sluggish, emotionally attached, and resistant to change. Meditation for Kapha should focus on energizing the mind and fostering mental clarity.

- **Dynamic Meditation**: Kapha types benefit from meditation practices that involve movement or energy, such as **Kundalini meditation** or **active visualization**. These practices engage the mind and body, helping to break up stagnant energy and boost vitality.
- **Breathing Techniques**: **Kapalbhati** (skull-shining breath) is an energizing pranayama technique that stimulates the digestive fire and clears congestion. By rapidly exhaling through the nose and inhaling passively, this breath helps to increase mental clarity, reduce lethargy, and energize the body.
- **Mindfulness Meditation**: For Kapha types, mindfulness meditation is an effective way to clear the mind and stay present. This technique involves paying attention to one's thoughts, feelings, and sensations in a non-judgmental way, which helps Kapha types avoid becoming overly attached or stuck in repetitive emotional patterns.

Meditation for Balancing All Doshas

Some meditation practices are universal and can benefit individuals of all doshic types by promoting overall well-being and balance. These techniques address both the mind and the body and can be practiced regularly to maintain a sense of harmony and peace.

- **Body Scan Meditation**: This technique involves mentally scanning the body, starting from the toes and moving up to the head, while focusing on relaxation and awareness of sensations in each part of the body. It helps to release physical tension and clear mental clutter, making it suitable for all doshas, especially when stress or anxiety is present.
- **Mantra Meditation**: Reciting a specific mantra helps align the mind with a higher frequency, promoting peace and balance. Simple mantras like **"Om"**, **"So Hum"**, or any calming phrase can help quiet the mind, reduce stress, and promote deep relaxation.
- **Chakra Meditation**: Focusing on the seven energy centers (chakras) in the body helps clear blockages and promote the free flow of prana. This practice balances all doshas and enhances mental, emotional, and spiritual health by aligning the body's energy centers with the mind.

The Importance of Consistency

In Ayurveda, meditation is not a one-time practice but a consistent, daily ritual that contributes to long-term health and balance. The benefits of meditation accumulate over time, creating a foundation for emotional resilience, mental clarity, and physical vitality. Just as Ayurveda emphasizes a balanced routine (**Dinacharya**) for daily living, meditation should be practiced regularly—ideally in the morning or evening—to integrate its calming, healing effects into everyday life.

Meditation is a powerful tool in Ayurveda for maintaining balance within the mind and body. By tailoring meditation practices to an individual's doshic constitution, Ayurveda encourages mental clarity, emotional stability, and spiritual growth. Whether through visualization, breathing techniques, or silent meditation, these practices help harmonize the doshas, clear mental toxins, and foster a deep connection to one's inner self. Incorporating meditation into daily life brings the body, mind, and spirit into alignment, promoting a healthier and more balanced existence.

Ayurvedic Daily Routine

In Ayurveda, a daily routine, or **Dinacharya**, is a key element for maintaining health and preventing disease. According to this ancient system of medicine, aligning your daily activities with the natural rhythms of your body, the environment, and the seasons helps balance the doshas (Vata, Pitta, and Kapha) and supports overall well-being. A well-structured daily routine promotes vitality, mental clarity, and emotional stability by harmonizing the body's internal processes with external influences like the time of day and seasonal changes.

Waking Up Early

The ideal time to wake up in Ayurveda is during the **Brahma Muhurta**, the period before sunrise, which occurs about 1.5 hours before dawn. This is considered the most auspicious time for spiritual practice, mental clarity, and physical rejuvenation. Waking up early allows you to tap into a peaceful, calm environment, free from the disturbances of the day. It is a time for self-reflection, meditation, and setting a positive tone for the day.

Hydration and Cleansing

After waking, it is important to hydrate the body. **Drinking warm water** with freshly squeezed lemon or a pinch of salt is recommended to flush out toxins that have accumulated overnight and to stimulate the digestive system. This helps balance **Vata**, **Pitta**, and **Kapha** by flushing out **Ama** (toxins) and stimulating the internal digestive fire (**Agni**).

Tongue scraping is another important Ayurvedic practice to remove toxins that have accumulated on the tongue overnight. This simple habit helps improve digestion and enhances taste perception.

Following tongue scraping, **oil pulling** (swishing oil in the mouth for several minutes) is recommended to detoxify the mouth, strengthen the teeth, and improve oral hygiene. **Sesame oil** or **coconut oil** are commonly used for this practice.

Morning Movement

Gentle exercise is an essential part of Ayurveda's daily routine. **Yoga** is particularly effective as it helps strengthen the body, calm the mind, and balance the doshas. **Vata** types benefit from grounding and stabilizing poses, **Pitta** types can focus on cooling and restorative movements, and **Kapha** types are encouraged to engage in dynamic, energizing practices. A morning walk or a short, gentle stretching session can also help stimulate circulation and boost energy levels for the day.

Abhyanga (Self-Massage)

Abhyanga, or self-massage with warm herbal oils, is an Ayurvedic practice that helps nourish the skin, improve circulation, and balance the doshas. **Vata** types should use **sesame oil** for its warming qualities, **Pitta** types benefit from **coconut oil** to cool the body, and **Kapha** types can use **mustard oil** for its stimulating properties. The practice of Abhyanga also calms the nervous system, reduces stress, and enhances lymphatic drainage.

Bathing

After self-massage, a warm bath or shower is recommended. Ayurveda suggests using natural soaps and oils to cleanse the skin, while also maintaining the body's moisture balance. A **warm shower** helps open the pores and removes toxins, while promoting relaxation.

Breakfast and Eating

Ayurveda recommends eating the largest meal of the day at **lunch**, as this is when digestion is strongest (around noon). However, a **light breakfast** is still essential to start the day. For a **Vata** type, warm, moist foods like oatmeal or porridge help ground and stabilize, while **Pitta** types benefit from cooling foods like fruit or yogurt. **Kapha** types may prefer lighter, stimulating foods such as fruits, warm herbal teas, or a small portion of nuts and seeds.

It is recommended to eat in a relaxed, mindful state, without distractions, to improve digestion. Avoid overeating and allow the body to focus on nutrient absorption and energy production.

Midday (Lunch)

Lunch should be the heaviest meal of the day, ideally eaten between 12 PM and 1 PM, when the digestive fire is at its peak. A well-balanced Ayurvedic lunch typically consists of **whole grains**, **vegetables**, **protein**, and **healthy fats**. **Vata** types should eat grounding, moist foods like soups or stews; **Pitta** types should have cooling, mildly spiced foods; and **Kapha** types benefit from light, stimulating meals with fewer oils and grains.

Afternoon Practices

After lunch, Ayurveda suggests taking a brief **rest** or a short walk. **Avoid strenuous exercise immediately after meals**, as it can disturb digestion. A light walk stimulates digestion, reduces stress, and supports detoxification.

In the afternoon, drinking **herbal teas** like **ginger**, **cinnamon**, or **peppermint** can help further stimulate digestion and balance the doshas. These teas also improve circulation, flush out toxins, and maintain energy levels throughout the day.

Evening Routine

As the evening approaches, Ayurveda recommends winding down with calming activities to promote restful sleep. **Avoiding heavy meals or caffeine in the evening** helps prepare the body for sleep. For **Vata** types, a **light dinner** is recommended around 6 PM, consisting of cooked vegetables and grains. **Pitta** types should focus on cooling foods, and **Kapha** types benefit from light, easily digestible meals.

Evening yoga or gentle stretching helps relax the body and ease any built-up tension from the day. **Pranayama** (breathing exercises), such as **Anulom Vilom** (alternate nostril breathing), helps calm the mind and release stress before bed.

Sleep

Ayurveda emphasizes the importance of a regular sleep schedule. The optimal time to sleep is between **10 PM and 6 AM**, aligning with the natural rhythms of the body and the environment. Sleep is considered essential for the body's restorative processes and for balancing the doshas. **Vata** types should aim to sleep early to avoid restlessness, **Pitta** types should ensure their sleeping environment is cool and calm, and **Kapha** types should focus on avoiding oversleeping and keeping the body energized during the day.

A daily routine in Ayurveda is more than a series of tasks; it is a lifestyle designed to maintain balance and support long-term health. By aligning your habits with the natural rhythms of your body and environment, you can achieve optimal vitality, mental clarity, and emotional stability. Whether through meditation, self-care practices, or mindful eating, Ayurveda's daily routine offers a path to well-being that nurtures the body, mind, and spirit. By adopting these principles into your life, you create a foundation for health, longevity, and inner peace.

Morning Rituals

In Ayurveda, the morning is considered the most important time of day for setting the tone for physical, mental, and emotional well-being. The early hours are seen as a time of renewal, where the body is naturally inclined to detoxify and rejuvenate. By following a structured morning ritual, or **Dinacharya**, individuals can align with the natural rhythms of the body and environment, helping to restore balance to the doshas (Vata, Pitta, and Kapha) and optimize digestion, energy, and mental clarity. Ayurveda emphasizes that a mindful morning routine enhances vitality, clears toxins, and sets the foundation for a healthy day ahead.

1. Wake Up Early

The best time to wake up in Ayurveda is during **Brahma Muhurta**, the 1.5-hour period before sunrise. This is considered a sacred time, optimal for spiritual practices, meditation, and setting a calm, focused mindset. Rising early allows you to take advantage of the peaceful, quiet atmosphere before the day's activities begin, promoting mental clarity and emotional calm. It is believed that waking up during this time enhances the natural energy flow and supports overall well-being throughout the day.

2. Hydration and Detoxification

After waking, it's important to rehydrate the body, as dehydration can cause sluggishness and hinder detoxification. **Drinking warm water** with freshly squeezed lemon or a pinch of salt is highly recommended. This simple practice helps flush out toxins (Ama) that have accumulated overnight and stimulates the digestive fire (**Agni**). Warm water is considered soothing to the digestive system and enhances nutrient absorption, preparing the body for the day ahead.

Tongue scraping is another Ayurvedic practice recommended in the morning. After sleep, the body naturally detoxifies, and a coating of toxins can accumulate on the tongue. Using a tongue scraper helps to remove this buildup, improving taste perception and stimulating the digestive system. This practice also promotes better oral hygiene and enhances overall digestion.

3. Oil Pulling

Oil pulling is an ancient Ayurvedic detoxifying technique that involves swishing oil (typically **sesame** or **coconut oil**) in the mouth for about 10-15 minutes. This practice helps remove bacteria and toxins from the mouth, strengthens the teeth, gums, and jaw, and improves oral hygiene. It is said to support overall detoxification and promote clear skin, as the oil draws out impurities from the body through the mouth.

4. Self-Massage (Abhyanga)

Abhyanga, or self-massage with warm herbal oils, is a rejuvenating practice that nourishes the skin, improves circulation, and balances the doshas. According to Ayurveda, massaging the body with oil helps to stimulate the lymphatic system, promote detoxification, and calm the nervous system. The type of oil used should align with your dosha:

- **Vata** types benefit from **sesame oil** for its grounding and warming qualities.
- **Pitta** types should use **coconut oil** for its cooling properties.
- **Kapha** types are suited to **mustard oil** for its stimulating effects.

Abhyanga not only helps detoxify the body but also reduces stress and promotes relaxation, leaving you feeling rejuvenated and balanced.

5. Meditation and Mindful Breathing

The early morning is the ideal time for **meditation** and **pranayama** (breathing exercises), which help to clear mental toxins, calm the mind, and set the intention for the day. Meditation practices such as **mindfulness meditation**, **mantra repetition**, or **guided visualization** promote focus, clarity, and emotional stability. These practices reduce stress, improve concentration, and cultivate a sense of inner peace.

Pranayama techniques such as **Nadi Shodhana** (alternate nostril breathing) or **Bhramari** (bee breath) are particularly beneficial. These practices enhance the flow of prana (life force) throughout the body, calm the nervous system, and help balance the doshas. They are especially effective for Vata and Pitta types, who may struggle with anxiety or overactive thoughts.

6. Light Physical Activity

After meditation, gentle movement is recommended to stimulate circulation and enhance energy. **Yoga** is particularly beneficial in the morning as it promotes flexibility, strengthens muscles, and calms the mind. Tailor your practice to your dosha type:

- **Vata types** should focus on grounding, slow-paced, and gentle stretches to stabilize their energy.
- **Pitta types** can benefit from cooling, restorative poses that help relax the mind and cool any internal heat.

- **Kapha types** benefit from more dynamic and invigorating yoga sequences that help boost energy and circulation.

In addition to yoga, a **morning walk** or a gentle stretching routine can help release tension, invigorate the body, and prepare the mind for the day ahead.

7. Cleanse and Refresh

After your morning self-care routine, it's time to refresh with a **warm shower** or bath. Ayurveda recommends using natural, non-toxic products like herbal soaps or oils to cleanse the skin and body. The warm water helps to open the pores, while the herbs or oils provide soothing and healing benefits for the skin and mind.

For Vata types, moisturizing after a shower is crucial to prevent dryness, while Pitta types may benefit from cooling herbal bath oils. Kapha types should avoid excessive moisture and instead focus on invigorating, energizing cleansers.

8. Nourishing Breakfast

Breakfast should be nourishing yet light, as it provides the first fuel for the body. Ayurveda recommends a **warm, easy-to-digest breakfast** that supports the digestive fire. For **Vata**, this means warm porridge or oatmeal with ghee and spices like cinnamon. **Pitta** types should enjoy cooling foods, such as fresh fruit, yogurt, or smoothies. **Kapha** types benefit from light, stimulating foods like herbal teas with a handful of nuts or seeds. Breakfast should be eaten mindfully, without distractions, to enhance digestion and promote balanced energy throughout the day.

9. Setting Intentions for the Day

As part of your morning ritual, take a moment to set positive intentions or practice gratitude. Reflecting on the day ahead, setting clear intentions, and aligning your actions with your values help foster a sense of purpose and mental clarity. This practice also allows you to approach the day with a sense of calm and focus, rather than rushing into the chaos of everyday tasks.

The Ayurvedic morning routine is designed to harmonize the mind, body, and spirit by following the natural rhythms of the day. By waking early, hydrating, practicing self-care rituals, meditating, and nourishing the body, you set the stage for a balanced and energetic day. These rituals not only cleanse the body of toxins but also ground the mind and promote emotional well-being, helping to maintain equilibrium in every aspect of life. By making these morning practices a consistent part of your routine, you create a foundation for long-term health, vitality, and inner peace.

Evening Practices

In Ayurveda, the evening is a time to wind down, restore balance, and prepare the body and mind for restful sleep. Just as the morning sets the tone for the day, the evening rituals play an essential role in promoting relaxation, improving digestion, and preventing the buildup of toxins (Ama). A mindful evening routine aligns with the body's natural rhythms, helping to harmonize the doshas (Vata, Pitta, and Kapha), clear mental clutter, and promote overall well-being.

1. Light Evening Meal

Ayurveda recommends having **dinner** at least two to three hours before bedtime to allow proper digestion before sleep. The evening meal should be light, warm, and easy to digest to avoid overburdening the digestive system. For **Vata** types, grounding, moist foods like soups or stews work well. **Pitta** types should focus on cooling, non-spicy dishes, such as vegetables, rice, or dairy. **Kapha** types benefit from light, easily digestible foods, like leafy greens or small portions of protein. It's best to avoid heavy, greasy, or spicy foods in the evening, as they can disrupt digestion and disturb sleep.

2. Herbal Teas for Digestion

Drinking **herbal teas** is a common Ayurvedic practice to enhance digestion and soothe the body before bedtime. **Chamomile**, **ginger**, **peppermint**, or **coriander tea** are particularly beneficial for evening use. These teas help calm the digestive system, relax the mind, and support the elimination of toxins from the body. **Triphala**, a blend of three fruits—**Amalaki**, **Bibhitaki**, and **Haritaki**—is often taken in small amounts at night to promote gentle detoxification and improve digestion.

3. Evening Yoga and Stretching

As the day winds down, **gentle yoga** can help release any built-up tension and calm the body and mind. Evening yoga sessions should focus on restorative, slow-paced postures that encourage relaxation, flexibility, and stress relief. For **Vata** types, gentle stretches and grounding poses like **Child's Pose** (Balasana) or **Legs Up the Wall** (Viparita Karani) help calm the nervous system. **Pitta** types should focus on cooling poses such as **Forward Bends** or **Seated Twists** to release heat and tension. **Kapha** types benefit from stimulating postures like **Spinal Twists** or **Standing Forward Bends** to counteract stagnation.

Breathing exercises like **Nadi Shodhana** (alternate nostril breathing) or **Bhramari** (bee breath) help calm the mind, reduce stress, and regulate the flow of energy in the body. These practices prepare the body for deep, restorative sleep.

4. Abhyanga (Self-Massage) with Warm Oils

Incorporating **Abhyanga**, or self-massage with warm oils, into the evening routine is an effective way to calm the nervous system and release physical tension. The oil used should align with your dosha type:

- **Vata** types benefit from **sesame oil**, which is grounding and warming.
- **Pitta** types should use **coconut oil** for its cooling and soothing properties.
- **Kapha** types can use **mustard oil** to stimulate circulation and invigorate the body.

Abhyanga not only nourishes the skin but also improves circulation, balances the doshas, and promotes relaxation, preparing the body for a restful sleep.

5. Digital Detox and Relaxation

Ayurveda encourages minimizing **stimulation** before bedtime to allow the mind and body to transition into a restful state. This includes reducing exposure to **blue light** from screens, such as smartphones, computers, or television. Instead, engage in relaxing activities such as reading, journaling, or spending quality time with family. Engaging in quiet, mindful activities encourages the parasympathetic nervous system to activate, helping to reduce stress and prepare the body for sleep.

6. Pranayama and Meditation

Pranayama, or controlled breathing, is an effective tool for calming the mind and reducing mental clutter in the evening. Techniques like **Ujjayi breath** (victorious breath) and **Anulom Vilom** (alternate nostril breathing) help bring focus and calmness to the mind. For those struggling with overactive thoughts or stress, these calming techniques are especially beneficial before bed.

Meditation is another valuable practice in the evening routine. Focusing on **mindfulness, guided imagery**, or **loving-kindness meditation (Metta)** helps relax the mind, reduce anxiety, and cultivate a sense of inner peace. Meditation enhances emotional well-being and promotes restful sleep by lowering the stress hormone cortisol and increasing levels of serotonin.

7. Creating a Restful Sleep Environment

According to Ayurveda, the **environment** plays a significant role in ensuring restful sleep. Ensure your bedroom is dark, quiet, and cool, as these factors support optimal sleep conditions. Avoid excessive noise or distractions, and maintain a temperature that promotes relaxation (generally cool for Pitta types and warm for Vata types).

For Pitta types, cooling essential oils such as **lavender** or **sandalwood** are beneficial for calming the mind before bed. **Vata** types can benefit from grounding scents like **frankincense** or **cedarwood**. Diffusing calming essential oils can help prepare the mind and body for sleep and ensure a restorative night.

8. Evening Reflection and Gratitude

Taking time to reflect on the day and practicing gratitude can help ease the transition from day to night. Ayurveda encourages individuals to mentally review the day's events with a sense of mindfulness and contentment. This practice of reflection reduces mental tension and emotional clutter, clearing the mind and creating a sense of peace. Writing down things you are grateful for or simply acknowledging your achievements and experiences for the day promotes emotional balance and enhances relaxation.

9. Sleep Routine

Ayurveda emphasizes a regular sleep schedule, with the ideal time to go to bed being between **10 PM and 6 AM**. This aligns with the body's natural circadian rhythm, which governs energy levels and detoxification processes. Going to bed at the same time each night ensures the body gets adequate rest and supports the rejuvenation of tissues and systems. For **Vata** types, it is especially important to go to bed early to maintain stability, while **Kapha** types should avoid oversleeping or napping during the evening to avoid feeling sluggish the next day.

Incorporating Ayurvedic practices into the evening routine helps the body unwind, detoxify, and rejuvenate for the night ahead. Whether through gentle yoga, breathing exercises, self-massage, or mindful reflection, these practices promote restful sleep, emotional balance, and overall well-being. A mindful evening routine not only enhances the quality of sleep but also supports long-term health by aligning the body's natural rhythms with the external environment. By embracing these Ayurvedic practices, individuals can experience deeper relaxation, better digestion, and a calmer, more centered mind.

Seasonal Routines in Ayurveda

In Ayurveda, **seasonal routines** are an integral aspect of maintaining balance and health. Just as the seasons change, so too do the energies in our bodies, and Ayurveda emphasizes the importance of aligning our lifestyle, diet, and self-care practices with the natural rhythms of nature. According to Ayurvedic principles, the qualities of each season directly affect the doshas (Vata, Pitta, and Kapha), and adapting to these shifts can prevent imbalance and disease. By following a seasonal routine, individuals can harmonize with the environment, enhance their vitality, and support overall well-being.

Winter: Warming and Grounding

In Ayurveda, **winter** is considered a time dominated by **Vata** dosha, which is associated with qualities like cold, dryness, and lightness. During this time, it is important to balance Vata's cold and dry qualities by focusing on warming, grounding practices. This season calls for nourishment, stability, and protection against the elements.

- **Diet**: Warm, moist, and oily foods are ideal for the winter months. Soups, stews, and cooked grains like rice and oats provide warmth and sustenance. Spices such as **ginger**, **cinnamon**, **cloves**, and **turmeric** stimulate digestion and help protect against the cold. Heavier, grounding foods like root vegetables, ghee, and healthy fats are recommended to provide stability and energy.
- **Self-care**: **Abhyanga** (self-massage with warm oil) is especially beneficial in winter, as it helps to nourish and hydrate dry skin, while also calming the nervous system. **Sesame oil** is ideal for Vata types, as it is warming and grounding. Additionally, **warm baths** and **steams** can help relieve dryness in the skin and joints, which are more prone to irritation during the colder months.
- **Lifestyle**: Winter is a time for rest and rejuvenation. It is important to get plenty of sleep to allow the body to rebuild energy reserves. Avoid excessive exposure to cold wind and drafts, and wear warm clothing to protect the body from the harsh weather. Gentle exercises like **yoga** and **walking** are beneficial for maintaining circulation without overexerting the body.

Spring: Detoxification and Renewal

Spring is associated with **Kapha** dosha, which embodies qualities like heaviness, moisture, and stability. As the weather shifts from cold to warm, the earth begins to thaw, and so too can excess moisture and stagnation accumulate in the body. Spring is a time for cleansing, detoxifying, and lightening up.

- **Diet**: The focus in spring should be on light, dry, and cooling foods that help reduce the excess moisture and heaviness of Kapha. Fresh fruits and vegetables, especially leafy greens, are perfect for this season. Foods like **asparagus**, **broccoli**, and **artichokes** help stimulate digestion and support detoxification. Avoid dairy, heavy grains, and fried foods, as they can exacerbate Kapha imbalances.
- **Self-care**: **Neti pots** (nasal irrigation) are often recommended to clear excess mucus and prevent sinus congestion, a common issue during the spring. **Abhyanga** with **mustard oil** or a stimulating herbal blend helps invigorate the body and clear stagnant energy. Regular exfoliation of the skin can also help clear out the buildup of toxins.
- **Lifestyle**: Spring is the season for renewal, so this is a great time to incorporate **detoxifying routines** into daily life. Consider a **gentle cleanse** or fasting routine, and take time to engage in activities that stimulate energy and creativity. Outdoor activities like hiking, cycling, or walking are especially beneficial, as they help to circulate the energy of the body and reduce Kapha's tendency toward sluggishness.

Summer: Cooling and Soothing

In **summer**, the dominant dosha is **Pitta**, which embodies qualities of heat, sharpness, and intensity. During the hot summer months, the body tends to accumulate excess heat, which can lead to irritability, inflammation, and dehydration. Ayurveda recommends focusing on cooling and calming practices to balance Pitta and avoid overheating.

- **Diet**: Summer calls for light, cool, and hydrating foods that help soothe internal heat. **Salads**, **cucumber**, **melon**, and **yogurt** are perfect choices for cooling the body. **Mint**, **coriander**, and **coconut** are also great cooling agents. Avoid spicy, salty, and fried foods, which can aggravate Pitta and increase internal heat. Hydration is key, so drink plenty of cool water, coconut water, or herbal teas such as **peppermint** or **chamomile**.
- **Self-care**: **Cool baths** or **showers** are highly beneficial in the summer to regulate body temperature and cleanse the skin. **Aloe vera** and **coconut oil** can be used to soothe the skin, especially if exposed to too much sun. **Abhyanga** with cooling oils, such as **coconut** or **sandalwood oil**, helps reduce Pitta heat and promotes relaxation.
- **Lifestyle**: During the summer, it is important to avoid overexposure to the sun, especially during midday when the heat is strongest. Take breaks throughout the day to relax in cool environments and engage in gentle, cooling activities such as

swimming or **yoga**. Ensure you get enough sleep, as excess heat can lead to restlessness and irritability, common signs of Pitta imbalance.

Fall: Grounding and Balancing

Fall is a transitional season that marks the shift from the warmth of summer to the cooler months of winter. It is a time when **Vata** dosha begins to dominate, as the qualities of dryness, coolness, and lightness become more prominent. Fall is a time to focus on grounding and nourishing the body to prepare for the winter months ahead.

- **Diet**: As the weather cools, incorporate warming, grounding, and nourishing foods into the diet. **Soups**, **stews**, and **root vegetables** like sweet potatoes, carrots, and squash help calm the dryness of Vata. Warm grains, like oats and quinoa, along with healthy fats such as ghee, are also recommended to support digestion and provide stability.
- **Self-care**: **Abhyanga** with warming oils, such as **sesame oil**, is highly beneficial in the fall, as it helps to moisturize the skin and calm the nervous system. Additionally, warm **herbal teas** like **ginger** or **cinnamon** can help stimulate digestion and promote circulation, alleviating the dry and cold qualities of Vata.
- **Lifestyle**: Fall is the season for reflection and preparation. This is a time to focus on creating a stable routine and nurturing the body with sufficient rest and relaxation. **Yoga** practices that emphasize grounding and centering, such as **forward bends** and **seated postures**, help soothe Vata and maintain physical and mental balance.

In Ayurveda, aligning your routine with the changing seasons ensures that the body stays in harmony with nature and that the doshas remain balanced throughout the year. By adapting your diet, self-care practices, and lifestyle according to the unique qualities of each season, you can optimize your health, prevent disease, and enhance vitality. Whether it's grounding in the winter, detoxifying in the spring, cooling in the summer, or balancing in the fall, seasonal routines in Ayurveda provide a holistic approach to living in tune with the natural world.

Ayurveda and Mental Health

In Ayurveda, mental health is considered an integral aspect of overall well-being, where the balance between the mind, body, and spirit is essential for a harmonious life. The ancient system of medicine recognizes that emotional and mental imbalances are often deeply connected to physical health, and vice versa. Ayurvedic practices aim to restore balance to the mind by addressing the root causes of mental disturbances, whether they stem from physical imbalances, poor digestion, stress, or emotional trauma. By understanding the interconnection between the doshas (Vata, Pitta, and Kapha), lifestyle choices, diet, and the mind, Ayurveda offers a holistic approach to promoting mental clarity, emotional stability, and mental resilience.

The Mind-Body Connection in Ayurveda

In Ayurveda, the mind and body are not separate entities but are intricately connected. The state of one directly influences the other. The **sattva**, **rajas**, and **tamas** qualities define the state of the mind. **Sattva** represents calmness, clarity, and purity; **rajas** embodies activity, restlessness, and desire; and **tamas** reflects dullness, lethargy, and confusion. Maintaining mental health involves cultivating **sattva** by reducing the influence of **rajas** and **tamas**. Ayurveda also links the mind's state to the doshas. When the doshas are in balance, the mind is calm, clear, and focused. However, when any dosha becomes aggravated, it can lead to mental disturbances like anxiety, depression, irritability, or emotional instability.

Mental Health and the Doshas

Each dosha influences mental and emotional tendencies, and understanding one's doshic constitution can provide insight into mental health patterns.

- **Vata**: The qualities of **Vata**—dryness, coldness, and lightness—are reflected in mental states that are often anxious, restless, and scattered. People with a dominant Vata dosha may experience feelings of overwhelm, fear, and instability. **Vata imbalance** can lead to anxiety, insomnia, and difficulty concentrating. To calm Vata, Ayurvedic practices emphasize grounding, routine, and warm, soothing foods. Meditation, calming breathing exercises like **Bhramari** (bee breath), and grounding yoga poses such as **Child's Pose** or **Tree Pose** can help stabilize the mind.

- **Pitta**: **Pitta** is associated with heat, intensity, and transformation. When **Pitta** is in balance, individuals tend to be focused, determined, and goal-oriented. However, when aggravated, Pitta can lead to irritability, frustration, anger, and stress. This imbalance may manifest as conditions such as perfectionism, burnout, or even rage. Cooling practices, like **Sitali** breath (cooling breath), gentle physical activities like swimming or walking, and cooling foods such as cucumbers and melons help to calm excess Pitta. Meditation practices focusing on relaxation and emotional release, as well as chanting, can be helpful in maintaining mental clarity and emotional balance for Pitta types.
- **Kapha**: **Kapha** is characterized by stability, calmness, and groundedness. While this dosha provides strength and endurance, when **Kapha** becomes imbalanced, it can lead to depression, lethargy, attachment, and emotional stagnation. Kapha imbalance may result in feelings of sadness, weight gain, and a tendency toward isolation. To balance Kapha, stimulating activities like aerobic exercise, engaging in new experiences, and incorporating spicy or warming foods like ginger and garlic are recommended. **Kapha** types may benefit from **Kapalbhati** (skull-shining breath) and **dynamic yoga** practices that help increase energy, clear mental fog, and uplift the mood.

Ayurvedic Practices for Mental Health

Ayurveda provides several holistic practices that promote mental well-being, all of which emphasize balance, routine, and connection to one's environment.

- **Diet**: Ayurveda recognizes the powerful effect of food on the mind. A diet that supports mental health should be light, nourishing, and easy to digest, as poor digestion can lead to the accumulation of **Ama** (toxins) and contribute to mental dullness or confusion. For instance, **Vata** types should eat grounding, warming foods to calm their anxious and scattered mind. **Pitta** types benefit from cooling and soothing foods to reduce their irritability and stress. **Kapha** types should focus on light, stimulating foods that boost energy and prevent stagnation. Additionally, foods high in antioxidants, healthy fats, and fresh vegetables are known to support mental clarity and emotional stability.
- **Herbal Remedies**: Ayurveda has a long tradition of using herbs to support mental health. **Ashwagandha**, an adaptogen, helps the body manage stress and anxiety by calming the nervous system and improving overall resilience. **Brahmi** (Gotu Kola) is another herb used to enhance cognitive function, clarity, and memory. **Tulsi** (Holy Basil) is revered for its ability to calm the mind, reduce stress, and support emotional balance. **Shankhapushpi** is known for its ability to enhance mental clarity and calm the mind, particularly for Vata imbalances.
- **Meditation and Pranayama**: Ayurveda emphasizes **meditation** as a powerful tool for achieving mental clarity and emotional stability. Meditation practices such as **mindfulness meditation** or **loving-kindness meditation** (Metta) cultivate

feelings of compassion, balance, and inner peace. **Pranayama** (breathing exercises) like **Nadi Shodhana** (alternate nostril breathing), **Bhramari** (bee breath), and **Ujjayi** (victorious breath) can calm the mind, reduce anxiety, and enhance concentration. These techniques help regulate prana (life force energy), balance the nervous system, and promote emotional harmony.
- **Sleep and Rest**: Proper rest and sleep are crucial for maintaining mental health. Ayurveda recommends an early bedtime (before 10 PM) to ensure deep, restorative sleep. For **Vata** types, regularity and warmth in the sleep environment are essential to avoid restlessness. **Pitta** types benefit from a cooling, calm environment, and **Kapha** types should avoid excessive sleep or naps to prevent sluggishness.

Lifestyle Practices for Mental Health

- **Routine and Balance**: Following a consistent daily routine (**Dinacharya**) is key to managing mental health. Ayurveda emphasizes waking up early, setting intentions for the day, and engaging in self-care practices like **Abhyanga** (self-massage) and yoga. A balanced routine helps stabilize the doshas, reduce stress, and foster emotional resilience.
- **Connection with Nature**: Ayurveda encourages individuals to spend time in nature, as it has a calming and healing effect on the mind. **Vata** types benefit from the grounding energy of nature, **Pitta** types from the soothing, cool qualities, and **Kapha** types from the invigorating, stimulating environment.

Ayurveda recognizes that mental health is not merely the absence of illness, but a dynamic state of balance and well-being. By addressing mental health through a combination of diet, lifestyle, self-care practices, and emotional balance, Ayurveda offers a holistic approach that nurtures the mind as much as the body. Understanding your dosha and implementing Ayurvedic practices tailored to your unique needs can help reduce stress, enhance mental clarity, and cultivate emotional stability, allowing for a healthier and more harmonious life.

Mind-Body Connection

In Ayurveda, the mind and body are seen as interconnected aspects of a person's overall health, each influencing the other in profound ways. This holistic approach recognizes that physical ailments often have mental or emotional roots, and vice versa. The Ayurvedic perspective on health emphasizes the balance between the physical body, the emotions, the mind, and the spirit. Achieving harmony in these areas is essential for maintaining well-being, and Ayurveda provides various tools, including diet, lifestyle practices, herbs, and meditation, to nurture this balance.

The Role of the Doshas

In Ayurveda, health is governed by the three primary energies or **doshas**—Vata, Pitta, and Kapha—which are responsible for all physiological and mental processes. Each dosha has specific qualities that affect both the body and the mind:

- **Vata** is linked to movement, change, and creativity. It governs the nervous system, circulation, and all bodily movements. Imbalance in Vata can lead to mental restlessness, anxiety, fear, and instability.
- **Pitta** is associated with transformation, digestion, and metabolism. It governs the body's heat and energy. Mentally, Pitta types are focused, determined, and intelligent, but when imbalanced, Pitta can lead to irritability, anger, frustration, and obsessive thoughts.
- **Kapha** is linked to structure, stability, and nourishment. It governs the body's tissues, strength, and immunity. When out of balance, Kapha can lead to feelings of heaviness, sadness, and lethargy, contributing to depression or emotional stagnation.

When these doshas are in harmony, both the body and mind function optimally. However, when one or more doshas become aggravated, it can lead to physical and emotional disturbances. For example, an excess of **Vata** may cause anxiety and digestive issues, **Pitta** imbalance may lead to irritability and inflammation, and **Kapha** imbalance could cause depression and weight gain. Ayurveda works to balance these doshas through diet, lifestyle, and natural remedies, promoting both physical and mental health.

The Importance of Agni (Digestive Fire)

In Ayurveda, **Agni**, or digestive fire, is a critical concept for maintaining both physical and mental health. Agni represents the body's ability to transform food into energy, and it also influences the mind's ability to process and assimilate thoughts. When Agni is strong, the body and mind are capable of digesting food, emotions, and experiences efficiently. However, when Agni is weak, it leads to poor digestion, toxin buildup (Ama), and mental fog. This imbalance manifests as lethargy, emotional instability, and physical ailments.

By balancing Agni through dietary choices, lifestyle habits, and herbal treatments, Ayurveda helps strengthen both the mind and body. For example, eating warm, easily digestible foods can promote a strong digestive fire, while meditation and pranayama (breathing exercises) can help calm the mind and reduce stress, improving the digestion of thoughts and emotions.

The Impact of Stress on the Body

Stress is one of the most common disruptors of the mind-body connection. In Ayurveda, it is believed that mental stress can manifest in physical ailments. Chronic stress can disturb the balance of the doshas, weaken the immune system, and impair digestion, leading to a variety of health issues such as headaches, digestive disturbances, high blood pressure, and skin problems.

Ayurveda recognizes the importance of **mental hygiene** and suggests practices like meditation, yoga, and breathing exercises to manage stress. These practices promote **sattva** (mental clarity and purity) and reduce **rajas** (mental agitation) and **tamas** (mental dullness), helping to restore balance and harmony in both the body and mind.

The Role of Emotions in Physical Health

In Ayurveda, emotions are seen as energies that can either flow freely or become trapped in the body, leading to disease. When emotions such as anger, fear, grief, or anxiety are suppressed or not processed properly, they can manifest physically as illness. For example, unresolved anger (a **Pitta** emotion) may lead to inflammatory conditions, while chronic worry and fear (often related to **Vata**) can cause digestive problems and anxiety.

Ayurveda offers various tools to release emotional blockages and promote mental health. Practices like **Abhyanga** (self-massage with warm oils), yoga, and meditation help to soothe the nervous system, release tension, and balance the emotions. **Herbs** like **Ashwagandha** (for stress), **Brahmi** (for mental clarity), and **Tulsi** (for emotional balance) are commonly used to support the mind-body connection and promote emotional resilience.

The Power of Mindfulness and Meditation

Ayurveda places a strong emphasis on mental wellness through practices like **meditation**, **mindfulness**, and **pranayama** (breathing exercises). These practices help calm the mind, increase self-awareness, and regulate emotions. Meditation, in particular, is a powerful tool for integrating the mind and body, allowing individuals to achieve emotional balance and mental clarity.

Mindfulness encourages individuals to be present in the moment, which reduces stress and fosters a deeper connection to both the body and mind. **Pranayama** practices, such as **Nadi Shodhana** (alternate nostril breathing), **Bhramari** (bee breath), and **Ujjayi** (victorious breath), help regulate the nervous system, calm the mind, and reduce the effects of stress and anxiety.

Ayurveda and the Five Senses

In Ayurveda, the five senses—**sight, smell, taste, touch,** and **hearing**—are considered powerful channels for influencing the mind and body. When the senses are overstimulated or not properly nourished, they can cause stress and imbalance. Ayurveda encourages practices that engage the senses in a balanced way to support mental and emotional health.

- **Sight**: Watching calming visuals, like nature scenes or soothing colors, can help calm the mind.
- **Smell**: Essential oils like lavender, sandalwood, and jasmine are used to reduce stress and promote mental clarity.
- **Taste**: Eating fresh, balanced foods tailored to one's dosha helps nourish the body and mind.
- **Touch**: Daily self-massage with warm oils (Abhyanga) is soothing for the nervous system and promotes mental clarity.
- **Hearing**: Listening to calming sounds, such as soft music or nature sounds, can promote relaxation and mental peace.

The mind-body connection in Ayurveda emphasizes the importance of balance in all aspects of life—physical, mental, and emotional. Through practices that nurture both the body and the mind, Ayurveda helps to restore harmony, reduce stress, and prevent illness. By following Ayurvedic principles such as a balanced diet, daily routines, meditation, and self-care, individuals can strengthen their mind-body connection, achieve emotional stability, and maintain overall health and vitality. In Ayurveda, true well-being arises from the harmonious relationship between the body, mind, and spirit.

Managing Stress with Ayurveda

In Ayurveda, stress is viewed as an imbalance in the body's energies, or **doshas**, which manifests both physically and emotionally. When the doshas are out of balance, they can lead to stress, anxiety, and other health issues. Ayurveda offers a holistic approach to managing stress by addressing the root causes of imbalance, strengthening the body's natural resilience, and promoting mental clarity. Through a combination of diet, lifestyle practices, herbal remedies, and mindful routines, Ayurveda provides powerful tools to manage stress and restore harmony between the body, mind, and spirit.

Understanding Stress and the Doshas

Each dosha—**Vata**, **Pitta**, and **Kapha**—reacts to stress in different ways. Understanding how each dosha is affected by stress can help guide treatment and lifestyle changes.

- **Vata**: Vata is associated with qualities like movement, dryness, and lightness. When Vata becomes aggravated by stress, it can lead to anxiety, restlessness, insomnia, and mental fatigue. Vata stress is often characterized by overthinking, worry, and a scattered mind.
- **Pitta**: Pitta governs transformation, heat, and intensity. Stress for Pitta types often manifests as frustration, irritability, anger, and perfectionism. They may become easily frustrated, burn out from overwork, or feel intense pressure to achieve their goals.
- **Kapha**: Kapha is linked to stability, structure, and calmness. However, when Kapha is imbalanced by stress, it can lead to feelings of stagnation, lethargy, depression, and attachment. Kapha types may become overwhelmed by emotional stress, feel sluggish, or develop a tendency to withdraw or become overly attached.

Ayurvedic Tools for Managing Stress

Ayurveda offers several practical tools to help manage stress, reduce its impact on the body, and restore balance to the mind and emotions.

1. Diet and Nutrition

In Ayurveda, the foods you eat are deeply connected to your mental and physical health. A balanced, nourishing diet helps maintain equilibrium and can support the body's natural ability to cope with stress. Specific dietary practices can be tailored to each dosha to help calm the mind and reduce stress.

- **Vata types** benefit from warm, grounding foods that calm their anxious, restless nature. Foods like cooked grains (rice, oats), soups, and stews, along with healthy fats (ghee, olive oil), provide stability and nourishment.
- **Pitta types** should focus on cooling, soothing foods to balance their fiery, intense energy. Avoid spicy, salty, or fried foods, and instead opt for salads, fresh fruits, dairy, and leafy greens to calm internal heat and reduce irritability.
- **Kapha types** should incorporate light, stimulating foods to reduce sluggishness and balance their tendency toward emotional attachment. Foods like bitter greens, legumes, and light grains like quinoa and barley help invigorate the body and mind.

In addition, incorporating **herbal teas** like **chamomile**, **ginger**, or **ashwagandha** can help calm the nervous system and promote relaxation. **Ashwagandha**, in particular, is a well-known adaptogen that helps the body adapt to stress, reduce anxiety, and improve overall resilience.

2. Breathing Techniques (Pranayama)

Breathing exercises are one of the most powerful Ayurvedic tools for managing stress. Pranayama (the practice of controlled breathing) helps to regulate the flow of prana (life force energy) through the body, calm the nervous system, and reduce mental agitation. Specific pranayama techniques can be tailored to each dosha to relieve stress and anxiety.

- **Vata**: For Vata types, **Nadi Shodhana** (alternate nostril breathing) is especially helpful in calming the nervous system, promoting mental clarity, and reducing feelings of anxiety or mental fog.
- **Pitta**: To cool excess heat and reduce frustration, **Sitali breath** (cooling breath) or **Ujjayi breath** (victorious breath) can be beneficial. These techniques help soothe the mind, reduce mental restlessness, and bring balance to Pitta.
- **Kapha**: For Kapha types, **Kapalbhati** (skull-shining breath) is an energizing pranayama that helps clear mental fog, increase alertness, and reduce emotional stagnation.

Daily pranayama practice can significantly reduce stress and improve mental clarity, helping individuals remain calm and centered in the face of challenges.

3. Meditation and Mindfulness

Meditation is a key practice in Ayurveda for managing stress and promoting mental health. It allows the mind to settle, reduces the impact of stress, and creates space for relaxation and introspection. Ayurveda recommends **mindfulness meditation**, where the practitioner focuses on the present moment without judgment. This practice helps reduce anxiety, improves emotional resilience, and promotes inner peace.

For **Vata** types, guided meditation or visualization is helpful, as it helps calm an overactive mind. For **Pitta**, **loving-kindness meditation** (Metta) can be used to reduce anger and frustration. **Kapha** types can benefit from dynamic meditation, which incorporates physical movement or visualization to energize the mind and release emotional stagnation.

4. Abhyanga (Self-Massage)

Abhyanga, or self-massage with warm oils, is an Ayurvedic practice that helps soothe the nervous system, promote circulation, and reduce stress. The act of massaging the body with oil calms the mind and alleviates tension in the muscles, making it an excellent practice for managing stress.

- **Vata types** benefit from **sesame oil**, which is grounding and warming, helping to reduce mental and physical dryness.
- **Pitta types** can use **coconut oil**, which cools and soothes the body, especially when experiencing excess heat or irritation.
- **Kapha types** are best suited to **mustard oil** or a stimulating herbal oil blend, which helps invigorate and energize the body.

This practice not only promotes relaxation but also enhances the circulation of prana, the life force energy, throughout the body, which helps to reduce stress and anxiety.

5. Adequate Sleep and Rest

In Ayurveda, **sleep** is considered one of the pillars of health, and its quality is closely linked to the body's ability to cope with stress. Ensuring that the body gets sufficient, restful sleep is vital for reducing stress and maintaining emotional balance. Ayurveda recommends going to bed by **10 PM**, as this is when the body is naturally inclined to rest and repair. A regular sleep routine helps stabilize the doshas and supports the body's ability to cope with the demands of daily life.

For **Vata** types, it is important to keep a consistent sleep schedule and create a warm, calming sleep environment. **Pitta** types should focus on cooling their bodies before bed, avoiding excessive stimulation, and creating a peaceful atmosphere. **Kapha** types should avoid oversleeping and ensure that their sleep is deep and refreshing.

6. Yoga and Physical Activity

Yoga is one of the most effective tools in Ayurveda for managing stress. The physical postures (asanas) help release tension from the body, improve circulation, and promote mental clarity. For stress relief, yoga should focus on calming, restorative poses.

- **Vata types** benefit from grounding and gentle yoga sequences that help settle the nervous system and promote relaxation, such as **Child's Pose** or **Seated Forward Fold**.
- **Pitta types** should focus on cooling and restorative poses, like **Forward Bends** and **Twists**, which calm internal heat and release frustration.
- **Kapha types** benefit from more dynamic movements that help release emotional stagnation and energize the body, such as **Sun Salutations** or **Standing Poses**.

Regular practice of yoga helps manage stress, improve flexibility, and enhance mental clarity, creating a sense of balance and well-being.

Managing stress with Ayurveda is a holistic approach that involves balancing the mind, body, and spirit. By incorporating diet adjustments, pranayama, meditation, self-care routines, and yoga into daily life, Ayurveda offers powerful tools to reduce stress, cultivate mental clarity, and promote emotional resilience. Ayurveda emphasizes that managing stress is not just about removing the symptoms but addressing the root causes, ensuring long-term health and harmony. By aligning with Ayurvedic principles, individuals can develop a deeper understanding of their unique stress triggers and create practices that help them maintain balance and well-being in all aspects of life.

Ayurvedic Treatments for Mental Disorders

In Ayurveda, mental health is closely tied to the balance of the body's energies, or doshas—**Vata**, **Pitta**, and **Kapha**. When these energies are out of balance, they can manifest as mental disorders such as anxiety, depression, insomnia, and stress. Ayurveda addresses mental health not only by treating the symptoms but by focusing on the root causes of mental and emotional disturbances. The Ayurvedic approach emphasizes the importance of diet, lifestyle changes, herbal remedies, and therapeutic treatments to restore balance, clarity, and emotional well-being.

Understanding Mental Disorders in Ayurveda

In Ayurveda, mental disorders are typically seen as imbalances in the **mind-body** connection. Mental stress and emotional instability are often linked to disruptions in the flow of **prana** (life force energy) through the body's energy channels (**nadis**) and the imbalance of the doshas. For instance:

- **Vata imbalances** can lead to feelings of anxiety, restlessness, and mental fatigue. This may manifest as nervousness, insomnia, and overactive thinking.
- **Pitta imbalances** often lead to irritability, frustration, anger, and perfectionism. Pitta types may experience emotional burnout, high stress, and intense emotions.
- **Kapha imbalances** are associated with depression, lethargy, and emotional stagnation. People with excessive Kapha may feel heavy, withdrawn, or mentally sluggish.

Ayurveda treats these mental health conditions by addressing the root cause of the imbalance, restoring harmony within the body's energies, and providing therapies to support the mind's clarity and peace.

Ayurvedic Treatments for Mental Disorders

1. **Herbal Remedies**

Herbs play a significant role in Ayurvedic treatments for mental health. Various plants are used to calm the mind, reduce stress, and restore emotional balance.

- **Ashwagandha**: This adaptogenic herb is well-known for its ability to combat stress and reduce anxiety. Ashwagandha supports the adrenal glands, calms the nervous system, and helps in emotional stabilization. It is often used to improve sleep, reduce mental fatigue, and alleviate symptoms of depression.
- **Brahmi (Gotu Kola)**: Brahmi is considered one of the best herbs for enhancing mental clarity, focus, and memory. It is particularly beneficial for anxiety and depression, as it promotes calmness and mental sharpness, making it ideal for Vata imbalances.
- **Tulsi (Holy Basil)**: Tulsi is a revered herb in Ayurveda for its ability to reduce stress, calm the mind, and enhance spiritual well-being. It is used to manage anxiety, nervousness, and emotional imbalances, particularly in Pitta and Kapha individuals.
- **Jatamansi**: This herb is known for its calming properties and is used to treat conditions like insomnia, anxiety, and stress. It helps to calm the mind and reduce nervous tension, especially when Vata is imbalanced.
- **Shankhapushpi**: A brain tonic, this herb is used to improve memory, focus, and cognitive function. It is often prescribed for individuals with mental fatigue or emotional instability, particularly in Kapha imbalances.

2. **Dietary Adjustments**

Diet is a central aspect of Ayurvedic treatment for mental health. Food influences the doshas and can either aggravate or calm mental disorders. To balance Vata, Pitta, and Kapha, Ayurveda recommends foods that soothe the mind and support digestive health.

- **Vata**: Since Vata is prone to dryness and irregularity, a Vata-pacifying diet includes warm, moist, grounding foods. **Cooked grains**, **soups**, and **steamed vegetables** help provide nourishment. Vata types should avoid raw foods and cold drinks, as they can increase anxiety and restlessness.
- **Pitta**: Pitta types benefit from cooling, soothing foods to calm their fiery nature. Foods like **cucumbers**, **yogurt**, and **leafy greens** help reduce internal heat. **Spicy and sour foods** should be avoided, as they can aggravate Pitta and lead to irritability and emotional burnout.
- **Kapha**: For Kapha types, a light and stimulating diet is necessary to prevent sluggishness and depression. **Spicy** foods, **legumes**, and **bitter greens** help balance Kapha by stimulating digestion and increasing energy. Kapha types should avoid heavy, sweet, and greasy foods that contribute to emotional stagnation.

In addition to foods, Ayurvedic nutrition emphasizes the importance of **eating mindfully**, chewing food thoroughly, and avoiding overeating. Regular meals at consistent times help maintain digestive fire (Agni) and emotional equilibrium.

3. **Pranayama (Breathing Exercises)**

Pranayama is one of the most effective Ayurvedic practices for managing stress and mental health. Breathing exercises help to calm the mind, regulate the nervous system, and reduce emotional turbulence. Specific pranayama techniques can help balance the doshas and alleviate symptoms of mental disorders.

- **Nadi Shodhana** (Alternate Nostril Breathing): This technique is particularly useful for calming Vata imbalances, as it helps reduce anxiety, promote mental clarity, and balance the nervous system.
- **Bhramari** (Bee Breath): Ideal for Pitta types, Bhramari helps to calm the mind, reduce stress, and lower levels of frustration and irritability. It is particularly effective for cooling excess heat and soothing an agitated mind.
- **Ujjayi** (Victorious Breath): Ujjayi is a soothing breath that helps calm both the body and mind. It is excellent for reducing stress, calming the nervous system, and promoting relaxation. It is especially beneficial for Pitta types who tend to have fiery emotions.

4. **Meditation and Mindfulness**

Meditation is a powerful Ayurvedic tool for reducing stress and cultivating mental balance. It allows individuals to clear mental clutter, achieve emotional stability, and improve overall mental clarity. Ayurveda recommends various forms of meditation based on an individual's dosha and emotional state.

- **Vata** types benefit from guided meditation or **visualization techniques** that help ground the mind and prevent overactive thinking.
- **Pitta** types should focus on **loving-kindness meditation** (Metta) or **breath-based meditation** to reduce anger, frustration, and stress.
- **Kapha** types may benefit from more dynamic or **energizing meditation** practices to overcome feelings of stagnation and promote emotional release.

Mindfulness practices, such as focusing on the present moment or practicing gratitude, can also be beneficial in reducing anxiety and depression, promoting mental resilience, and fostering emotional well-being.

5. **Daily Routine and Lifestyle Practices**

A consistent daily routine, or **Dinacharya**, is an important aspect of Ayurvedic treatment for mental health. Establishing a structured routine helps calm Vata, reduce stress, and promote emotional stability. A daily routine includes practices like waking up early, eating at regular intervals, and engaging in activities like yoga, meditation, and self-care.

Abhyanga (self-massage with warm oil) is also recommended for mental health, as it nourishes the body, calms the nervous system, and promotes emotional grounding. A regular practice of Abhyanga helps reduce stress and supports the body's natural detoxification processes, which can improve both physical and mental health.

6. **Therapeutic Treatments**

For individuals experiencing more severe mental imbalances, Ayurveda recommends **Panchakarma**, a comprehensive detoxification and rejuvenation program. Panchakarma therapies, including **Virechana** (purgation), **Basti** (enema therapy), and **Shirodhara** (oil pouring on the forehead), help cleanse the body of toxins, improve mental clarity, and restore balance to the doshas. These treatments are often combined with other Ayurvedic practices to help alleviate symptoms of anxiety, depression, and other mental disorders.

Ayurveda provides a holistic and personalized approach to mental health, addressing the underlying causes of mental disorders rather than merely treating symptoms. By restoring balance to the doshas through diet, herbs, breathing exercises, meditation, and lifestyle practices, Ayurveda helps individuals achieve mental clarity, emotional stability, and overall well-being. This comprehensive approach to mental health emphasizes the interconnectedness of the body, mind, and spirit, offering a path to healing that is both effective and sustainable.

Ayurveda and Sleep

In Ayurveda, sleep is considered a cornerstone of health, closely linked to the body's natural cycles and its ability to repair and rejuvenate. The ancient system views sleep as essential for balancing the doshas (Vata, Pitta, and Kapha), restoring energy, and promoting mental clarity. Quality sleep is thought to contribute not only to physical vitality but also to emotional and spiritual well-being. Ayurveda recognizes that poor sleep patterns or imbalances in sleep can lead to both physical and mental disturbances, which in turn can affect the doshas and overall health.

The Role of the Doshas in Sleep

Each dosha affects sleep in different ways, and understanding how they influence sleep can help tailor practices to promote restorative rest.

- **Vata**: Vata is the dosha of movement, and when it becomes imbalanced, it can lead to restlessness, anxiety, and insomnia. Individuals with a dominant Vata may experience disturbed sleep due to their overactive minds, frequent waking, or difficulty falling asleep. To balance Vata and promote restful sleep, grounding practices are essential. A warm, calming bedtime routine, warm baths, and the use of grounding herbs like **ashwagandha** or **chamomile** can help calm the nervous system and prepare the body for sleep.
- **Pitta**: Pitta governs metabolism and transformation, and when out of balance, it can result in difficulty winding down or a tendency to stay mentally alert late into the night. Pitta imbalances can lead to intense thoughts, irritability, and overheating, all of which disrupt sleep. To soothe Pitta and encourage restful sleep, cooling activities and calming practices are recommended. **Sitali breath** (cooling breath) before bed, a cool room temperature, and soothing herbal teas like **mint** or **lavender** help calm the mind and body, promoting a peaceful night's rest.
- **Kapha**: Kapha, associated with stability and heaviness, tends to lead to long, deep sleep, but when imbalanced, it can cause excessive sleep, lethargy, and difficulty waking in the morning. Kapha types may struggle with oversleeping or feeling sluggish upon waking. To balance Kapha, stimulating activities, such as light exercise or **Kapalbhati** (skull-shining breath), are recommended during the day. A lighter evening meal and avoiding excessive sleep during the day can also help regulate Kapha's tendency toward excess rest.

Ayurvedic Practices for Better Sleep

Ayurveda offers several practical recommendations for improving the quality of sleep based on an individual's constitution and doshic imbalances. These practices help to calm the mind, balance the doshas, and promote deep, restorative rest.

1. **Establish a Consistent Sleep Routine**
   Ayurveda emphasizes the importance of a regular sleep schedule. Going to bed and waking up at the same time each day aligns with the body's natural circadian rhythms, helping to strengthen the body's internal clock. Ideally, bedtime should be between **10 PM and 6 AM**, as this period aligns with the body's natural detoxification and rejuvenation processes. Early bedtime supports the healing of **Vata** and **Pitta**, while maintaining Kapha balance.
2. **Create a Calming Bedtime Routine**
   To ease the transition into sleep, Ayurveda recommends engaging in relaxing activities before bed. **Abhyanga**, a self-massage with warm oil, is particularly beneficial in calming Vata and Pitta and preparing the body for rest. **Sesame oil** is often recommended for Vata types to ground and nourish, while **coconut oil** is suitable for Pitta types to cool the body. Practicing **gentle yoga** or **meditation** before bed can also calm the mind, reduce stress, and prepare the body for deep rest.
3. **Herbal Remedies for Sleep**
   Ayurvedic herbs are frequently used to support healthy sleep and promote relaxation. **Ashwagandha**, an adaptogen, helps to regulate the body's stress response and support restful sleep. **Brahmi** (Gotu Kola) is another herb that calms the mind and supports mental clarity, while **chamomile** and **lavender** are known for their calming properties. Drinking **warm milk with turmeric** or **spiced milk** (made with cinnamon, cardamom, or saffron) before bed can also promote relaxation and induce sleep, especially for Vata and Pitta types.
4. **Dietary Considerations for Sleep**
   What you eat plays a key role in your ability to sleep well. Ayurveda recommends a light evening meal at least two hours before bedtime to allow for proper digestion. Foods that are grounding and easy to digest are ideal for promoting sleep. For **Vata types**, warm, moist foods like soups, stews, or cooked grains are ideal. **Pitta types** should avoid spicy, oily, or acidic foods, instead favoring cooling, hydrating foods like leafy greens, cucumbers, and dairy. **Kapha types** benefit from lighter meals with less sugar and fewer fats, focusing on foods that stimulate digestion without weighing them down.

Certain foods, such as **warm dairy** (like warm milk or ghee), **bananas**, **almonds**, and **oats**, are known to promote the release of **serotonin**, a precursor to **melatonin**, the hormone responsible for regulating sleep. Avoid heavy, rich, or stimulating foods before bedtime, as they can disturb digestion and keep the body in a state of heightened activity.

5. **Breathing Techniques and Pranayama**
   Breathing exercises can help calm the nervous system and promote deep relaxation before sleep. Pranayama techniques, such as **Nadi Shodhana** (alternate nostril breathing), **Bhramari** (bee breath), or **Ujjayi** (victorious breath), are effective for reducing stress, calming the mind, and promoting restful sleep. Breathing exercises encourage the flow of prana (life force) and balance the doshas, helping to clear mental clutter and create a peaceful mental state conducive to sleep.
6. **Sleep Environment**
   The environment in which you sleep plays a crucial role in Ayurveda. To promote restful sleep, it is important to create a calming, comfortable space. The bedroom should be cool, dark, and quiet, with minimal distractions. For **Pitta types**, a cool room is essential to reduce heat buildup, while **Vata types** may benefit from a warm, cozy space that provides grounding. Essential oils like **lavender**, **sandalwood**, or **frankincense** can be diffused to create a soothing atmosphere. A peaceful, relaxing environment helps ease the transition into sleep and encourages deep, restorative rest.

Ayurveda's View on Sleep Disorders

Ayurveda views sleep disorders as a result of doshic imbalances, poor lifestyle choices, or emotional stress. For example, **insomnia** is often linked to an excess of **Vata** or **Pitta**, while excessive sleepiness or lethargy can result from **Kapha** imbalance. Treatment for sleep disorders typically involves a combination of dietary changes, herbal remedies, pranayama, meditation, and lifestyle adjustments to restore harmony and balance to the mind and body.

For those struggling with chronic sleep issues, Ayurvedic treatments such as **Panchakarma** (a detoxification process) may be recommended to cleanse the body of accumulated toxins and restore internal balance. **Shirodhara**, a therapy involving the pouring of warm oil on the forehead, is another Ayurvedic treatment known to promote deep relaxation and help with sleep disturbances related to stress or anxiety.

In Ayurveda, sleep is viewed as essential for restoring balance, rejuvenating the body, and maintaining mental clarity. By aligning lifestyle practices with the natural rhythms of the body and focusing on diet, herbal remedies, pranayama, and creating a calming environment, Ayurveda offers a comprehensive approach to improving sleep quality. Understanding your unique doshic constitution and addressing any imbalances with personalized Ayurvedic practices can help you achieve restful, restorative sleep and maintain overall health and well-being.

Ayurvedic Sleep Rituals

In Ayurveda, sleep is considered a vital aspect of overall health, and establishing a calming nighttime routine is key to ensuring restful, rejuvenating sleep. Ayurvedic sleep rituals are designed to align with the body's natural rhythms, promoting relaxation, balancing the doshas, and preparing the mind and body for deep, restorative rest. These rituals emphasize calming practices that support the nervous system, regulate digestive fire (Agni), and clear any mental or emotional clutter that might interfere with a peaceful night's sleep.

1. Establish a Consistent Sleep Schedule

Ayurveda emphasizes the importance of routine, particularly when it comes to sleep. Going to bed and waking up at the same time each day helps regulate the body's internal clock and supports overall doshic balance. According to Ayurvedic principles, the ideal time for sleep is between **10 PM and 6 AM**, which aligns with the body's natural circadian rhythms and its rejuvenating processes. Waking up early, ideally before sunrise, allows for a peaceful, grounded start to the day and sets the tone for rest at night.

2. Create a Relaxing Bedtime Routine

A soothing pre-sleep routine is essential for calming both the body and mind. Ayurveda suggests engaging in calming activities before bed to promote deep relaxation. These activities help reduce stress and mental restlessness, particularly for those with Vata imbalances, which often lead to anxiety and sleeplessness.

- **Abhyanga (Self-Massage)**: A warm oil self-massage with **sesame oil** (for Vata) or **coconut oil** (for Pitta) is one of the most recommended Ayurvedic sleep rituals. Abhyanga helps calm the nervous system, promote circulation, and release muscle tension, making it easier to transition into sleep. It also provides nourishment to the skin, which can be particularly beneficial during the colder months or for dry skin conditions.
- **Herbal Bath**: A warm bath infused with calming herbs like **lavender**, **chamomile**, or **sandalwood** helps to relax both the body and mind. The warmth of the water relaxes the muscles, while the herbs calm the senses, promoting a state of tranquility. Bathing before bed helps prepare the body for rest and supports the purification process, soothing any accumulated stress.
- **Aromatherapy**: Using **essential oils** such as **lavender, sandalwood**, or **frankincense** in a diffuser or as a pillow spray can create a peaceful, soothing

environment. Aromatherapy has long been used in Ayurveda to calm the mind and relieve tension, making it easier to fall asleep.

3. Mindful Eating and Drinking

Ayurveda encourages a light evening meal that is easy to digest, as heavy or spicy foods can disrupt sleep. A light meal, such as **kitchari** (a nourishing blend of rice and lentils) or a warm vegetable soup, helps to ease digestion without burdening the body before sleep.

It's also recommended to avoid caffeine, alcohol, and excessive sugar in the evening, as they can interfere with the body's ability to unwind. **Warm herbal teas** like **chamomile**, **ashwagandha**, or **licorice root** are excellent choices to support relaxation and promote restful sleep. These herbs have calming properties and help soothe the digestive system, which is especially important for Vata and Pitta types who may experience stress or indigestion before bed.

4. Pranayama (Breathing Techniques)

Breathing exercises, or **pranayama**, are powerful tools in Ayurveda for preparing the mind and body for sleep. These techniques help to calm the nervous system, reduce stress, and bring balance to the doshas.

- **Nadi Shodhana** (Alternate Nostril Breathing) is particularly effective for calming the mind, reducing anxiety, and improving mental clarity. This practice helps balance Vata, which is often responsible for mental restlessness and insomnia.
- **Bhramari** (Bee Breath) is another excellent technique for reducing tension and stress. By making a gentle humming sound while exhaling, this pranayama helps calm the mind, reduce mental chatter, and prepare the body for restful sleep.
- **Ujjayi** (Victorious Breath) is a calming, deep breathing practice that helps soothe the body, slow the heart rate, and promote relaxation. Ujjayi breath is particularly helpful for those with Pitta imbalances, which can cause an overstimulated mind and body before sleep.

5. Meditation and Relaxation Techniques

Meditation is a cornerstone of Ayurvedic practice and is highly effective in promoting restful sleep. Incorporating meditation into your nightly routine helps quiet the mind, reduce emotional disturbances, and create a deep sense of inner peace.

- **Mindfulness Meditation**: Focus on your breath or practice body scanning to relax tension in the body and release stress. This type of meditation helps cultivate awareness in the present moment and reduce the racing thoughts that often keep the mind active at night.

- **Guided Meditation**: Using calming sounds or visualizations can be a helpful tool for people with Vata imbalances, who often experience overactive minds. Guided meditations, such as imagining a peaceful scene or journey, can help relax the mind and prepare it for sleep.
- **Loving-Kindness Meditation (Metta)**: This meditation focuses on cultivating feelings of love, compassion, and kindness toward oneself and others. It's particularly useful for Pitta types, who may experience frustration or anger, as it helps to soften the emotions and bring peace.

6. Creating the Ideal Sleep Environment

Creating a sleep-friendly environment is crucial for supporting deep and restful sleep. Ayurveda recommends the following environmental adjustments:

- **Cool Room for Pitta**: If you're a Pitta type, ensure your room is cool and well-ventilated to reduce the heat that can cause restlessness and irritability. A cooler room temperature can help lower internal body temperature and calm the mind.
- **Cozy Space for Vata**: Vata types benefit from a warm and cozy environment, which provides grounding and stability. Use soft, warm blankets, and ensure the room is free of drafts to avoid Vata's tendency toward coldness and restlessness.
- **Quiet and Darkness**: A quiet, dark environment is essential for sleep. Ayurveda recommends using blackout curtains or sleep masks to block out excess light and noise. Avoid using electronic devices before bed, as the blue light emitted can interfere with the production of melatonin, the sleep hormone.

7. Timing of Sleep

In Ayurveda, the ideal time to go to bed is before **10 PM**, as this aligns with the body's natural rhythms. Sleep is considered most restorative during the Kapha time of day, between **10 PM and 2 AM**, when the body's energy is naturally inclined to rest and repair. Avoid staying up late, as it can disturb the natural flow of the doshas and lead to physical and emotional imbalance.

Ayurvedic sleep rituals are designed to nurture the body, calm the mind, and restore balance to the doshas. By incorporating grounding practices such as warm self-massage, calming teas, breathing exercises, and meditation, you can promote deep, restorative sleep that rejuvenates both body and mind. Adapting these rituals to your doshic constitution ensures that your sleep environment and practices align with your unique needs, setting the stage for optimal health and vitality.

Ayurvedic Remedies for Sleep Disorders

In Ayurveda, sleep disorders are viewed as imbalances in the body and mind that disrupt the natural rhythm of rest and rejuvenation. Ayurveda recognizes that the quality of sleep is closely linked to the balance of the doshas (Vata, Pitta, and Kapha), and disturbances in any of these energies can lead to issues such as insomnia, restless sleep, or excessive drowsiness. By addressing the root causes of these imbalances—whether through diet, herbal remedies, lifestyle practices, or mental relaxation techniques—Ayurveda offers a holistic approach to managing and treating sleep disorders.

Understanding Sleep Disorders in Ayurveda

Ayurveda believes that imbalances in **Vata**, **Pitta**, and **Kapha** doshas can manifest in various sleep disturbances:

- **Vata imbalance** can lead to restlessness, anxiety, and difficulty falling asleep. Vata types may have a scattered, racing mind that prevents them from achieving deep, restful sleep.
- **Pitta imbalance** often results in the inability to wind down, with Pitta types experiencing mental intensity, frustration, and overheating, which can cause insomnia or disturbed sleep.
- **Kapha imbalance** tends to result in excessive sleep or feelings of sluggishness, lethargy, and difficulty waking up in the morning. Kapha types may also feel mentally foggy upon waking, even after a full night's rest.

Ayurvedic treatments focus on restoring balance to the doshas, calming the nervous system, and promoting mental and physical relaxation to address the root causes of sleep disorders.

Ayurvedic Remedies for Sleep Disorders

1. Herbal Remedies

Herbs play a central role in Ayurvedic treatment for sleep disorders. They help calm the mind, balance the doshas, and promote relaxation.

- **Ashwagandha**: This adaptogenic herb is commonly used in Ayurveda to reduce stress and anxiety, which are often underlying causes of sleep disorders. It helps balance Vata by calming the nervous system, promoting deep sleep, and improving overall resilience to stress.
- **Brahmi (Gotu Kola)**: Known for its ability to enhance mental clarity, Brahmi also has calming properties. It's especially beneficial for Pitta types, helping to cool an overheated mind and reduce mental agitation that may interfere with sleep.
- **Jatamansi**: This herb is particularly useful for calming an overactive mind and promoting restful sleep. It is known for its ability to alleviate anxiety, stress, and mental restlessness, making it ideal for people suffering from insomnia due to Vata imbalances.
- **Chamomile**: Often used as a mild sedative, chamomile helps to reduce stress and promote sleep by calming the nervous system. Drinking chamomile tea before bed can help prepare the body and mind for restful sleep.
- **Tulsi (Holy Basil)**: Tulsi is known for its adaptogenic properties, which help the body adapt to stress. It also supports the nervous system and promotes mental clarity, making it an excellent herb for Pitta types who may experience emotional heat or mental agitation that interferes with sleep.

2. **Pranayama (Breathing Exercises)**

Breathing exercises are an effective Ayurvedic remedy for calming the nervous system and promoting deep relaxation, essential for overcoming sleep disorders.

- **Nadi Shodhana** (Alternate Nostril Breathing): This pranayama technique is highly beneficial for calming the mind and balancing Vata. It helps reduce anxiety, clears mental clutter, and promotes mental clarity and relaxation, making it easier to fall asleep.
- **Bhramari** (Bee Breath): Bhramari is an excellent technique for soothing the mind and relieving tension. It is particularly helpful for Pitta types who may experience intense thoughts or frustration before sleep. The humming sound helps calm the nervous system and reduces stress, making it easier to relax into sleep.
- **Ujjayi** (Victorious Breath): This breathing technique creates a calming effect on the mind and is especially helpful for reducing anxiety and tension. Ujjayi helps release stress and promotes relaxation by slowing the breath and bringing awareness to the present moment.

3. **Dietary Adjustments**

In Ayurveda, the food you consume significantly impacts your sleep quality. A diet that supports digestive health and balances the doshas can help alleviate sleep disturbances.

- **Vata types** should eat grounding, warm foods to balance the dry, light qualities of Vata. Warm soups, stews, and cooked grains like rice or oats are ideal. **Vata types** should avoid cold, dry foods and caffeine, which can increase anxiety and disrupt sleep.
- **Pitta types** benefit from cooling foods that calm the internal heat. Foods such as cucumbers, leafy greens, and dairy products like milk or yogurt help cool the body and mind. Avoiding spicy, oily, and fried foods before bed is key to ensuring a peaceful night's rest.
- **Kapha types** should focus on light, stimulating meals in the evening to avoid sluggishness and oversleeping. A light, easily digestible meal with vegetables, legumes, and whole grains is ideal. **Kapha types** should avoid heavy, oily foods and excess sugar, as they can lead to lethargy and disturbed sleep patterns.

Additionally, drinking warm milk with **turmeric** or **saffron** before bed can promote relaxation and improve sleep quality. **Herbal teas** like chamomile or **valerian root** can also be soothing and helpful in preparing for rest.

4. **Self-Care Practices**

Ayurveda places a strong emphasis on self-care as a way to reduce stress and promote relaxation. **Abhyanga**, the practice of self-massage with warm oil, is one of the best ways to prepare the body for sleep. Abhyanga helps calm Vata by grounding the body and calming the nervous system.

- **Sesame oil** is typically recommended for Vata and Kapha types, as it is grounding and nourishing. **Coconut oil** is more suitable for Pitta types due to its cooling properties. Massaging the scalp with warm oil can also help to soothe the mind and promote restful sleep.

5. **Sleep Environment**

Creating a peaceful, relaxing environment is crucial for enhancing sleep quality. Ayurveda suggests that the sleep environment should support the body's natural rhythms and promote balance.

- For **Vata** types, a warm, cozy environment with soft, calming lighting can help soothe the nervous system. Using a humidifier or placing a warm water bottle in bed can also help relieve dryness and promote comfort.
- **Pitta types** benefit from a cool, quiet, and well-ventilated room. Keeping the room temperature low and using calming scents such as **lavender** or **sandalwood** can help cool internal heat and promote relaxation.

- **Kapha types** should aim to avoid excessive sleep, as they tend to oversleep or feel sluggish upon waking. A clean, well-organized space with a sense of lightness and openness can help reduce emotional stagnation and encourage better sleep quality.

6. **Panchakarma Therapy**

For individuals with chronic or severe sleep disorders, Ayurveda recommends **Panchakarma**, a detoxification therapy that includes practices like **Virechana** (purgation), **Basti** (enemas), and **Shirodhara** (pouring warm oil on the forehead). These treatments help detoxify the body, release accumulated stress, and restore balance to the doshas, ultimately improving sleep quality.

Shirodhara, in particular, is highly effective for insomnia and anxiety, as it calms the nervous system and promotes deep relaxation. This therapy can be done in conjunction with other Ayurvedic treatments to address the root causes of sleep disturbances.

Ayurveda offers a comprehensive and holistic approach to managing sleep disorders by focusing on the root causes of imbalance and promoting overall wellness. Through a combination of herbal remedies, pranayama, dietary adjustments, self-care practices, and creating the right environment for sleep, Ayurveda provides natural solutions for improving the quality of sleep. By addressing doshic imbalances and fostering relaxation, Ayurvedic remedies can restore healthy sleep patterns and support mental and physical well-being.

Sleeping Positions in Ayurveda

In Ayurveda, the way you sleep is just as important as the quality of your sleep. Ayurvedic principles suggest that your sleeping position can directly influence the balance of the doshas (Vata, Pitta, and Kapha) and affect your overall health and well-being. Sleep positions are believed to impact energy flow in the body, influence digestion, and either support or disrupt the natural alignment of the mind and body. By adopting the right sleeping position for your doshic constitution, you can promote better rest, reduce stress, and improve digestion and mental clarity.

Vata and Sleep Positions

Vata is associated with qualities such as dryness, lightness, and movement. Vata types are generally more prone to restlessness, anxiety, and insomnia. Their active, often scattered minds can lead to difficulty falling asleep or staying asleep. To help calm Vata imbalances, Ayurveda recommends sleeping in a position that supports grounding, stability, and relaxation.

- **Best Position**: **Sleeping on the left side** is most beneficial for Vata types. This position helps balance the flow of energy in the body, especially the movement of **prana** (life force energy), and promotes digestive health. Sleeping on the left side encourages better lymphatic drainage and facilitates the proper flow of bile, which can improve digestion and detoxification. Additionally, this position is soothing for the nervous system and helps calm an overactive mind.
- **Other Recommendations**: If sleeping on the left side is uncomfortable, Vata types can also sleep on their **back** with a **pillow under their knees**. This position supports the natural curves of the spine, reduces tension, and encourages deep relaxation. To enhance comfort and grounding, using **warm blankets** or **cozy pillows** can help reduce Vata's tendency to feel cold and restless at night.

Pitta and Sleep Positions

Pitta is the dosha of heat, intensity, and transformation. Pitta types are often determined, focused, and goal-oriented, but when out of balance, they can become irritable, frustrated, and overheated. To support Pitta's natural calm and bring down excessive internal heat, Ayurveda recommends sleeping in positions that allow the body to cool down and reduce stress.

- **Best Position**: **Sleeping on the right side** is ideal for Pitta types, as it helps reduce the flow of excess heat and promotes overall cooling. The right side encourages the proper functioning of the liver, the organ associated with Pitta, and supports detoxification processes. This position is particularly helpful for those who experience nighttime acidity, heartburn, or anger-related disturbances.
- **Other Recommendations**: Pitta types should also avoid sleeping on their stomachs, as it can aggravate heat in the body and lead to neck or back tension. **Sleeping on the back** with a cooling pillow or using a **soft mattress** can provide adequate support and help Pitta types relax more easily, especially if they experience mental overactivity or frustration before bed.

Kapha and Sleep Positions

Kapha is associated with qualities of heaviness, stability, and moisture. Kapha types are generally calm, patient, and slow-moving but may experience lethargy, depression, or excessive sleep when out of balance. To maintain balance and reduce Kapha's tendency toward sluggishness or emotional stagnation, Ayurveda recommends sleeping positions that invigorate and stimulate energy.

- **Best Position**: **Sleeping on the left side** is also beneficial for Kapha types. This position helps stimulate the digestive system and ensures the proper flow of lymphatic fluid, which aids in detoxification. Since Kapha's energy can sometimes become stagnant, this position helps increase circulation and reduces the feeling of heaviness or congestion, especially in the chest or abdomen.
- **Other Recommendations**: **Sleeping on the back** with a **slightly elevated head** can also be helpful for Kapha types, as it prevents excess heaviness and congestion in the chest and promotes clear breathing. This position supports the respiratory system and can help reduce the tendency to oversleep or feel sluggish upon waking.

General Ayurvedic Guidelines for Sleep Positions

While specific sleep positions may benefit each dosha differently, Ayurveda also provides some general recommendations that apply to everyone for enhancing sleep quality:

- **Sleep on a Firm Mattress**: Ayurveda recommends sleeping on a firm mattress, as this helps support the spine's natural alignment and promotes restful sleep. A soft or overly plush mattress may disrupt posture and lead to discomfort or stiffness, especially for Vata types.
- **Pillow Position**: The head should be supported with a pillow that promotes proper alignment of the spine. For **Vata**, a thicker pillow that supports the neck's natural curve is ideal. For **Pitta**, a thinner pillow may be preferable to avoid excess heat

around the head. **Kapha types** may find a medium pillow height best to maintain balance without feeling too heavy or restricted.
- **Avoid Sleeping on the Stomach**: Ayurveda generally advises against sleeping on the stomach, as this can create pressure on the internal organs, particularly the digestive system, and disrupt the natural flow of energy in the body. This position may also strain the neck and back, leading to discomfort.
- **Establish a Sleep Routine**: Ayurveda stresses the importance of consistency in sleep schedules. Going to bed at the same time each night and waking up at the same time each morning helps stabilize the doshas and regulate the body's circadian rhythm. This routine is particularly beneficial for those with **Vata** imbalances, as it promotes grounding and relaxation before sleep.

Enhancing Sleep with Ayurvedic Practices

Along with the ideal sleep positions, Ayurveda recommends several practices to promote restful and rejuvenating sleep:

- **Abhyanga (Self-Massage)**: Regular self-massage with warm oil can relax the body, calm the mind, and promote deep, restorative sleep. Using **sesame oil** (for Vata), **coconut oil** (for Pitta), or **mustard oil** (for Kapha) can balance the doshas and prepare the body for rest.
- **Herbal Teas**: Drinking calming herbal teas such as **chamomile, ashwagandha**, or **turmeric** before bed can help reduce stress and improve sleep quality. These herbs support relaxation, reduce anxiety, and soothe the nervous system.
- **Meditation and Pranayama**: Meditation and breathing exercises like **Nadi Shodhana** (alternate nostril breathing) or **Bhramari** (bee breath) can calm the mind, release stress, and prepare the body for sleep. Practicing these techniques regularly before bed can help create a peaceful transition into rest.

In Ayurveda, the sleep position you choose can significantly impact your overall health and well-being. By aligning your sleeping posture with your doshic constitution and adopting calming nighttime routines, you can improve the quality of your sleep, support digestion, and restore balance to your mind and body. Through mindful adjustments to sleep positions, as well as complementary Ayurvedic practices, you can create an environment conducive to restful, rejuvenating sleep and enhance your health in the long term.

Ayurveda for Women

In Ayurveda, women's health is considered a unique and holistic experience that encompasses not only the physical body but also emotional, mental, and spiritual well-being. Ayurveda views women as deeply connected to nature's cycles, with their health influenced by factors such as hormonal balance, menstrual cycles, pregnancy, childbirth, and menopause. By understanding the interplay between the body's doshas (Vata, Pitta, and Kapha) and aligning lifestyle, diet, and self-care practices with their individual needs, Ayurveda offers a natural, personalized approach to promoting health and vitality for women at all stages of life.

Dosha Balance for Women's Health

In Ayurveda, a woman's health is influenced by the balance of her doshas, which are combinations of the five elements (earth, water, fire, air, and ether). The doshas determine physical characteristics, mental tendencies, and overall energy levels. The doshic balance may shift throughout a woman's life, and Ayurveda provides personalized guidelines to address specific health needs at each stage.

- **Vata** is the dosha of movement and governs the nervous system, circulation, and elimination. Vata imbalances often manifest as anxiety, dryness, irregular periods, and fatigue. Women with a predominance of Vata may experience mental restlessness or emotional instability, especially around menopause or in the postpartum period.
- **Pitta** governs metabolism, digestion, and transformation. It regulates body heat, digestion, and energy. Pitta imbalances in women often lead to issues like inflammation, skin conditions (such as acne), and irritability, particularly around menstruation or pregnancy.
- **Kapha** is the dosha of stability and structure. Kapha is responsible for lubrication, immunity, and growth. When Kapha is out of balance, women may experience weight gain, lethargy, and excess mucus, particularly during pregnancy or in the later stages of life.

Understanding a woman's dominant dosha or any imbalances in these energies is key to creating a balanced lifestyle and a personalized treatment plan.

Ayurvedic Practices for Hormonal Balance

Ayurveda considers women's hormonal cycles to be deeply connected to their doshic balance, and it provides specific recommendations to support the body during different stages of hormonal change, including menstruation, pregnancy, and menopause.

1. **Menstrual Health** Ayurveda promotes a healthy menstrual cycle by focusing on digestive health (Agni), reducing stress, and balancing the doshas. Proper diet and lifestyle can support regular, pain-free menstruation. For example:
    - **Vata imbalances** can cause irregular or painful periods, as well as mood swings. To balance Vata, women should eat grounding, warm foods and focus on rest, avoiding excessive activity or stress.
    - **Pitta imbalances** may lead to heavy bleeding, irritability, or inflammation. Cooling foods and herbs, such as **mint** or **coconut**, along with calming practices like meditation, can help soothe Pitta.
    - **Kapha imbalances** may result in sluggish menstruation and weight gain. Stimulating exercises and light, detoxifying foods can help reduce Kapha's heaviness.
2. **Pregnancy and Postpartum Care** During pregnancy, Ayurveda focuses on nourishment, maintaining energy, and supporting emotional well-being. Women are encouraged to eat a warm, nurturing diet, rich in healthy fats, protein, and whole grains, to build strength and vitality. Specific herbs such as **Shatavari**, known for its ability to balance the female reproductive system, are often recommended to enhance fertility and support the health of both the mother and child.

    After childbirth, the postpartum period is considered a time of healing and rejuvenation. Ayurveda emphasizes rest, gentle exercise, and a healing diet that supports lactation and recovery. **Ghee**, **warm broths**, and **spices like ginger and turmeric** are typically included to nourish the body, restore energy, and promote mental clarity. Ayurvedic massage and herbal baths also help soothe and restore the body's natural balance.

3. **Menopause** Menopause is a natural transition in a woman's life, but it can also bring challenges such as hot flashes, mood swings, and sleep disturbances. Ayurveda helps women manage these changes by balancing the doshas and supporting the body's natural processes.
    - For **Pitta imbalances** during menopause, cooling foods, herbs like **Shatavari**, and practices like **pranayama** (breathing exercises) can help manage heat, reduce irritability, and promote emotional balance.
    - **Vata** imbalance during menopause can cause dryness, anxiety, and sleeplessness. Grounding foods, gentle yoga, and calming herbs like **ashwagandha** and **Brahmi** can help soothe Vata and support restful sleep.

- **Kapha imbalances** may cause weight gain, lethargy, or emotional stagnation. A stimulating diet, regular exercise, and detoxifying herbs can help prevent Kapha from becoming excessive during this time.

Ayurvedic Diet for Women's Health

The Ayurvedic approach to diet emphasizes eating for one's dosha, incorporating seasonal foods, and maintaining balance in digestion. A personalized, nourishing diet supports women's hormonal health and overall vitality.

- **Vata-pacifying foods** are grounding and moisturizing. Warm soups, stews, whole grains, and root vegetables are ideal for Vata types, especially during the colder months. Foods like **avocado**, **ghee**, and **almonds** help nourish Vata, prevent dryness, and improve digestion.
- **Pitta-pacifying foods** are cooling and hydrating. Pitta types should focus on fresh fruits and vegetables, especially cucumbers and leafy greens, and avoid spicy, sour, or oily foods that may increase internal heat.
- **Kapha-pacifying foods** are light and stimulating. **Spices** like ginger, turmeric, and garlic, along with **legumes** and **bitter greens**, help stimulate digestion and prevent Kapha imbalances, particularly when weight gain or sluggishness is an issue.

Ayurveda also recommends eating meals at regular intervals, avoiding heavy or processed foods, and using herbs such as **Triphala** to support digestion and elimination.

Ayurveda for Emotional Health

Ayurveda recognizes that emotional well-being is an essential part of women's health. Hormonal fluctuations, life transitions, and societal pressures can all influence a woman's emotional state. Ayurveda encourages practices that foster mental clarity, emotional resilience, and inner peace.

- **Meditation and mindfulness** help reduce stress, increase emotional awareness, and cultivate a sense of balance.
- **Yoga** practices that focus on flexibility and relaxation, such as gentle stretches or restorative poses, help release emotional tension stored in the body, calm the mind, and improve circulation.
- **Pranayama (breathing exercises)**, such as **Bhramari** (bee breath) or **Nadi Shodhana** (alternate nostril breathing), help balance the nervous system, reduce anxiety, and increase mental focus.

Ayurvedic Beauty and Self-Care

Self-care is an essential part of Ayurvedic health for women. Ayurveda encourages daily rituals to nourish the body, maintain vitality, and enhance beauty. Practices like **Abhyanga** (self-massage with warm oils), regular **detoxification**, and using **herbal face masks** or **moisturizing oils** promote healthy skin, hair, and overall well-being.

Herbs like **Amla** and **Neem** are used for skin health, while **Brahmi** and **Shankhapushpi** are recommended for mental clarity and emotional balance. Ayurvedic self-care rituals encourage women to listen to their bodies, connect with nature, and nourish themselves holistically.

Ayurveda offers a personalized, balanced approach to women's health that takes into account the body, mind, and spirit. By focusing on the doshas, adopting seasonal and lifestyle-based practices, and using natural remedies, women can support their hormonal health, emotional well-being, and overall vitality throughout the various stages of life. Through the wisdom of Ayurveda, women can experience a deeper sense of connection to themselves, their bodies, and their natural cycles, promoting long-term health, balance, and vitality.

Ayurveda and Female Health

In Ayurveda, female health is viewed through a holistic lens, where the body, mind, and spirit are seen as interconnected and equally important in maintaining well-being. The health of women is deeply influenced by their unique physiological and emotional needs, which are shaped by their hormonal cycles, life stages, and lifestyle. Ayurveda offers personalized guidance and natural remedies to address common concerns such as menstrual health, fertility, pregnancy, menopause, and emotional balance. The goal is not just to treat symptoms, but to restore balance to the body's energies (doshas), promote vitality, and support long-term wellness.

The Role of the Doshas in Female Health

In Ayurveda, health is maintained when the three doshas—**Vata**, **Pitta**, and **Kapha**—are in harmony. Each dosha governs different physiological functions, and an imbalance in one or more can impact a woman's health, particularly in the areas of hormonal regulation, digestion, mood, and reproductive health.

- **Vata** governs movement, the nervous system, and the elimination process. Women with a predominant Vata constitution may be more prone to anxiety, irregular menstrual cycles, dryness, or insomnia. Balancing Vata through grounding practices and a nourishing diet is key to maintaining emotional and physical stability.
- **Pitta** is associated with transformation, heat, and digestion. Women with a Pitta imbalance may experience conditions such as inflammation, PMS, acne, or hot flashes, especially around menstruation or menopause. Cooling foods, stress management, and cooling herbs like **Shatavari** can help soothe the fiery nature of Pitta.
- **Kapha** is linked to structure, stability, and lubrication. Women with a dominant Kapha dosha may have more stable moods and body structure but can be prone to weight gain, sluggish digestion, or lethargy. Kapha imbalances may also affect emotional well-being, leading to feelings of stagnation or depression.

Balancing the doshas with diet, lifestyle, and herbal remedies tailored to individual needs is central to Ayurvedic care for women's health.

Menstrual Health and Ayurveda

In Ayurveda, the menstrual cycle is closely connected to the doshas and the overall balance of the body's energies. A regular and symptom-free cycle is considered a sign of health, while imbalances may manifest in various forms, including painful periods (dysmenorrhea), irregular cycles, heavy bleeding, or mood swings. Ayurveda focuses on balancing the doshas, supporting digestive fire (Agni), and maintaining proper detoxification.

- **Vata imbalances** may lead to irregular cycles, dryness, or pain. Vata types are encouraged to maintain a warm, grounding routine, avoid excessive exercise, and consume nourishing, moist foods.
- **Pitta imbalances** can cause irritability, anger, or heavy bleeding. Cooling foods such as cucumbers, coconut, and leafy greens, along with calming activities like meditation, can help balance Pitta.
- **Kapha imbalances** may result in a sluggish cycle, with excessive bleeding or water retention. Kapha types should eat light, stimulating foods and engage in regular physical activity to encourage circulation and prevent stagnation.

Herbal remedies such as **Shatavari**, **Turmeric**, and **Ginger** are commonly used in Ayurveda to regulate menstrual health, reduce inflammation, and support overall reproductive function.

Fertility and Pregnancy

Ayurveda views fertility as the ability to create balance, not only physically but emotionally and spiritually. The health of a woman's **reproductive system** is influenced by factors such as digestion, circulation, emotional well-being, and hormonal balance. **Vata** imbalances can affect fertility by disrupting the flow of energy and nourishment to the reproductive organs, while **Pitta** imbalances can lead to inflammation or hormonal disruptions.

- **Shatavari**, known for its role in balancing female hormones, is often used to support fertility. It tonifies the reproductive system, balances hormones, and promotes overall vitality.
- **Ashwagandha** is another herb used to reduce stress and promote reproductive health. It is particularly beneficial for balancing Vata and Pitta, which can interfere with conception if out of balance.

During pregnancy, Ayurveda emphasizes the importance of nourishing the body with warm, easily digestible foods, while avoiding cold or heavy foods that can disrupt digestion. Herbal preparations like **Raspberry Leaf** and **Ginger** are often used to support digestion, ease nausea, and strengthen the uterus.

Menopause and Ayurveda

The transition into menopause can be a time of profound physical and emotional changes, as the body shifts away from the reproductive phase and hormone levels fluctuate. Ayurveda approaches menopause as a natural process, where the focus is on maintaining balance and promoting vitality, rather than viewing it as a disorder.

- **Pitta types** may experience hot flashes, irritability, and skin issues due to the increased heat in the body. Cooling foods, herbs like **Shatavari** and **Aloe Vera**, and calming practices like **yoga** and **pranayama** are beneficial for managing these symptoms.
- **Vata types** may face dryness, anxiety, and sleep disturbances as hormonal fluctuations disrupt the nervous system. Grounding activities, moisturizing oils, and nourishing foods like **ghee** and **avocado** can help balance Vata during this transition.
- **Kapha types** may experience weight gain, lethargy, or emotional stagnation. Light, stimulating foods and regular exercise can help regulate Kapha energy and prevent stagnation during menopause.

Ayurvedic herbs like **Ashwagandha** and **Brahmi** are often recommended to help reduce stress, support cognitive function, and improve overall well-being during menopause.

Ayurvedic Lifestyle Practices for Women's Health

In addition to diet and herbs, Ayurveda places great emphasis on lifestyle practices that support a woman's health, particularly in relation to managing stress, maintaining digestion, and promoting hormonal balance.

- **Abhyanga (self-massage)** is a rejuvenating practice that helps women maintain physical and mental balance. Daily self-massage with warm, dosha-specific oils promotes relaxation, reduces stress, and improves circulation.
- **Yoga and Pranayama** (breathing exercises) are essential for balancing the body and mind. Yoga helps with flexibility, circulation, and emotional release, while pranayama techniques such as **Nadi Shodhana** (alternate nostril breathing) and **Bhramari** (bee breath) calm the nervous system, reduce anxiety, and improve sleep quality.
- **Adequate Rest and Sleep**: Ayurveda stresses the importance of sleep in maintaining hormonal balance and emotional stability. A regular sleep schedule, ideally between **10 PM and 6 AM**, is essential for women to rejuvenate the body and mind.

Ayurvedic Beauty and Self-Care

Ayurveda also integrates beauty practices that promote glowing skin, healthy hair, and overall vitality. **Turmeric**, **Neem**, and **Amla** are commonly used for skincare and to promote detoxification. For women experiencing stress or hormonal imbalances, a calming skincare routine using **rose water** or **sandalwood oil** can help soothe and nourish the skin.

Daily self-care rituals like **Abhyanga** (self-massage with warm oils), regular detoxification, and the use of natural beauty products help women maintain not only physical health but emotional well-being.

Ayurveda offers a comprehensive, individualized approach to female health by addressing the physical, emotional, and spiritual aspects of a woman's life. Through personalized diet, lifestyle practices, herbal remedies, and treatments, women can achieve balance and vitality at every stage of life. Whether it is managing menstrual health, supporting fertility, navigating menopause, or promoting emotional well-being, Ayurveda provides the tools to help women live in harmony with their bodies and nature, supporting long-term health and wellness.

Ayurvedic Pregnancy Care

In Ayurveda, pregnancy is seen as a sacred and transformative period where the health and well-being of the mother directly influence the development of the baby. Ayurveda emphasizes holistic care during pregnancy, addressing not just physical health but also emotional and spiritual balance. The goal is to support the mother in maintaining vitality, emotional harmony, and mental clarity, while also promoting the healthy development of the baby. Ayurvedic practices during pregnancy focus on nourishing the body, strengthening the immune system, reducing stress, and creating a balanced environment for both mother and child.

The Importance of Dosha Balance During Pregnancy

Pregnancy can cause shifts in the doshas (Vata, Pitta, and Kapha), leading to specific symptoms and discomforts. Ayurveda recommends aligning diet, lifestyle, and self-care practices to balance the doshas and support the changing needs of the body. Each stage of pregnancy may call for different doshic support:

- **Vata imbalance** during pregnancy can cause dryness, anxiety, and discomfort in the lower abdomen. Women experiencing Vata imbalance may also feel mentally scattered or emotionally unstable. To soothe Vata, Ayurveda recommends warm, grounding foods and regular self-care practices like oil massage and rest.
- **Pitta imbalance** can result in increased heat, irritability, and inflammation, often leading to conditions like heartburn or skin rashes. Cooling foods and herbs such as **coconut** and **mint**, along with stress-reducing practices, can help balance Pitta and keep emotional heat in check.
- **Kapha imbalance** during pregnancy is often characterized by lethargy, weight gain, and sluggish digestion. Kapha types benefit from light, stimulating foods and moderate exercise to keep energy levels high and prevent emotional stagnation.

Diet and Nutrition for Pregnancy

In Ayurveda, diet is fundamental to the health of both the mother and the baby. Pregnancy is considered a time when the digestive fire (Agni) is crucial, as it ensures proper absorption of nutrients and supports overall vitality.

- **Nourishing, easily digestible foods** are emphasized throughout pregnancy. Warm, cooked foods such as **soups**, **stews**, **rice**, **lentils**, and **vegetables** support healthy digestion and nourishment for both mother and baby.
- **Whole grains** like **oats**, **quinoa**, and **rice** are recommended, as they provide a steady source of energy and stabilize blood sugar levels. **Healthy fats**, such as **ghee**, **avocado**, and **nuts**, are vital for fetal development, particularly for the brain and nervous system.
- **Protein-rich foods** such as **mung beans**, **tofu**, and **lentils** provide the building blocks necessary for growth. **Fresh fruits** like **apples**, **pears**, and **pomegranates** provide essential vitamins and antioxidants, which support immune function and skin health.
- **Hydration** is equally important. Women should drink warm water or **herbal teas** such as **ginger** or **chamomile** to stay hydrated and promote digestion.

Ayurvedic diet also suggests eating in a calm, mindful way, avoiding overeating, and making mealtimes a peaceful ritual. **Frequent, smaller meals** are recommended to keep the digestive fire strong and avoid discomfort.

Herbal Support During Pregnancy

Ayurvedic herbs offer natural remedies to support the body's changes during pregnancy. However, it's important to use herbs under the guidance of a qualified Ayurvedic practitioner to ensure their safety and effectiveness.

- **Shatavari** is one of the most commonly used herbs in Ayurveda for women's reproductive health. It helps balance hormones, supports the uterus, and promotes overall fertility. Shatavari is known for its ability to calm Vata and nourish the female reproductive system during pregnancy.
- **Ginger** is beneficial for digestion, helping to prevent nausea and improve appetite. It is especially useful during the first trimester when morning sickness is common.
- **Turmeric** is often used for its anti-inflammatory properties and ability to promote digestion and circulation. It also supports the immune system and helps balance Pitta during pregnancy.
- **Ashwagandha** helps reduce stress and anxiety, which can be particularly beneficial during pregnancy. It is also a natural adaptogen, promoting overall vitality and strengthening the immune system.
- **Amla** (Indian gooseberry) is a powerful antioxidant that helps nourish the skin and boost immunity, while also enhancing the absorption of nutrients.

Lifestyle Practices for Pregnancy

Alongside diet and herbs, Ayurveda recommends specific lifestyle practices to promote well-being during pregnancy. These practices focus on relaxation, emotional balance, and physical health.

1. **Abhyanga (Self-Massage)**: Daily self-massage with warm **sesame oil** (for Vata) or **coconut oil** (for Pitta) helps calm the nervous system, improve circulation, and prevent the discomfort of pregnancy, such as swelling, muscle cramps, or dry skin. Regular massage also promotes relaxation, which is essential for reducing stress.
2. **Yoga and Exercise**: Gentle yoga is highly beneficial for pregnant women. Specific yoga poses focus on flexibility, strength, and relaxation, particularly in the hips and pelvis, to support the body's changing needs. Breathing exercises (pranayama) like **Nadi Shodhana** (alternate nostril breathing) and **Bhramari** (bee breath) help reduce anxiety and promote mental clarity.
3. **Rest and Sleep**: Adequate rest and sleep are crucial during pregnancy to support the body's rejuvenation and energy reserves. Ayurveda emphasizes going to bed early, ideally before **10 PM**, to align with the body's natural circadian rhythms. Women should aim to create a peaceful and restful sleep environment.
4. **Mindfulness and Emotional Well-Being**: Pregnancy can bring about emotional fluctuations, and Ayurveda encourages mindfulness practices such as meditation, deep breathing, and affirmations to support emotional well-being. Women are advised to avoid excess stress and engage in activities that foster calmness, joy, and positive thinking.
5. **Hydrotherapy**: Warm water baths or foot soaks with Epsom salts or essential oils such as **lavender** or **sandalwood** can be soothing, reduce swelling, and promote relaxation. A warm bath before bed is a great way to unwind.

Preparing for Labor and Postpartum Care

Ayurveda also focuses on preparing the body for labor and ensuring a smooth recovery postpartum. In the weeks leading up to delivery, some Ayurvedic practices include:

- **Perineal massage** with **warm sesame oil** to prepare the body for labor, improve circulation, and prevent tearing.
- **Gentle herbal tonics** like **Shatavari** can be used in the third trimester to strengthen the uterus and prepare it for childbirth.

Postpartum care in Ayurveda is considered a time of rest, rejuvenation, and deep nourishment. The first 40 days after childbirth are seen as crucial for recovery. Ayurveda recommends:

- **Warm, nourishing foods** like soups, **ghee**, and **broths** to replenish energy and nourish breast milk production.
- **Restorative self-care practices** such as continued **Abhyanga** and rest to support recovery and prevent emotional imbalances like postpartum depression.
- **Herbal teas** such as **fenugreek** or **fennel** to support lactation and digestion.

Ayurvedic pregnancy care is based on a personalized, holistic approach that addresses the physical, emotional, and spiritual needs of the mother and child. By focusing on the balance of the doshas, providing nourishment, and incorporating mindful practices, Ayurveda helps women maintain vitality, reduce stress, and support the healthy development of their babies. Through a combination of diet, herbs, self-care, and relaxation, Ayurvedic practices offer a natural and nurturing way to navigate the journey of pregnancy and childbirth with ease, joy, and balance.

Ayurveda and Menopause

In Ayurveda, menopause is viewed as a natural transition in a woman's life, marking the end of her reproductive years and the beginning of a new phase of wisdom and vitality. Rather than being seen as a disorder or something to be feared, Ayurveda treats menopause as an opportunity for rejuvenation, personal growth, and the cultivation of inner balance. The approach is holistic, considering the physical, emotional, and spiritual changes women experience during this time. By restoring harmony to the doshas (Vata, Pitta, and Kapha) and supporting the body's natural rhythms, Ayurveda offers a personalized framework for managing the symptoms of menopause while promoting overall health.

The Role of the Doshas During Menopause

During menopause, the body undergoes significant hormonal changes, which can lead to imbalances in the doshas, particularly **Vata**. Vata, which governs movement, dryness, and change, becomes more prominent during this stage. The transition may bring about symptoms such as hot flashes, dryness, irritability, mood swings, and sleep disturbances. Understanding the influence of the doshas during menopause helps guide Ayurvedic treatments that address both the symptoms and the underlying imbalances.

- **Vata**: The onset of menopause is associated with an increase in Vata energy, which is responsible for change, dryness, and instability. Women experiencing a Vata imbalance during menopause may feel anxious, mentally scattered, and physically restless. They may also experience dryness in the skin, hair, and mucous membranes, as well as irregularities in digestion and sleep.
- **Pitta**: The intensity of Pitta energy can cause symptoms like hot flashes, irritability, skin rashes, and digestive issues. Women who have a predominantly Pitta constitution may notice a more pronounced impact of heat, leading to emotional imbalances such as frustration and anger.
- **Kapha**: As Kapha is the dosha of structure and stability, its influence during menopause may manifest as weight gain, emotional stagnation, or feelings of heaviness. Women with a predominance of Kapha may experience symptoms such as sluggishness, fatigue, and a tendency to withdraw emotionally.

By understanding these doshic imbalances, Ayurveda recommends specific dietary, lifestyle, and herbal practices to restore harmony during menopause and ease the transition.

Ayurvedic Approaches to Menopause Symptoms

1. **Dietary Recommendations**

In Ayurveda, food is considered medicine, and during menopause, diet plays a critical role in balancing the doshas and managing symptoms.

- **For Vata**: Grounding, nourishing foods are essential. Warm, moist, and easily digestible foods like **soups**, **stews**, and **whole grains** help calm the dryness and irregularity that Vata tends to bring. Foods rich in healthy fats, such as **ghee**, **avocado**, and **nuts**, nourish the body and help reduce the internal dryness that can be exacerbated during menopause.
- **For Pitta**: Cooling foods are vital to balance the heat of Pitta. **Cucumbers**, **leafy greens**, **coconut**, and **dairy** are helpful in cooling down the body and reducing inflammation. It is also important to avoid spicy, salty, or oily foods, which can exacerbate the heat and lead to irritability and hot flashes.
- **For Kapha**: Kapha-balancing foods are light, stimulating, and detoxifying. A diet rich in **bitter greens**, **legumes**, and **spices** like **ginger** and **turmeric** can help stimulate digestion and metabolism, prevent weight gain, and support mental clarity.

Ayurveda also recommends avoiding caffeine and alcohol, which can destabilize Vata and Pitta energies and disrupt sleep patterns. Instead, **herbal teas** like **chamomile**, **ginger**, or **peppermint** are ideal for calming the mind and supporting digestion.

2. **Herbal Remedies**

Ayurvedic herbs are commonly used to manage the symptoms of menopause. They support hormonal balance, ease emotional upheavals, and promote physical vitality.

- **Shatavari**: This herb is considered a cornerstone of Ayurvedic treatment for female reproductive health. Shatavari helps to nourish and balance the female reproductive system, regulate hormonal fluctuations, and ease symptoms like hot flashes, dryness, and mood swings. It is particularly beneficial for Vata and Pitta types during menopause.
- **Ashwagandha**: Known for its adaptogenic properties, ashwagandha helps the body adapt to stress and reduces anxiety, fatigue, and insomnia. It also strengthens the immune system and supports the overall vitality of the body, making it an excellent herb during the transition of menopause.
- **Brahmi**: This herb is known for its ability to calm the nervous system, improve mental clarity, and reduce anxiety and stress. Brahmi supports cognitive function and helps reduce the emotional instability that can occur during menopause.

- **Amla (Indian Gooseberry)**: Rich in antioxidants, Amla supports the immune system, enhances energy levels, and promotes healthy skin. It is often used to combat the fatigue and dryness that many women experience during menopause.

3. **Self-Care Practices**

Ayurveda emphasizes the importance of self-care during menopause to support mental, emotional, and physical health. These practices help promote relaxation, grounding, and balance.

- **Abhyanga (Self-Massage)**: Daily self-massage with warm oils helps reduce Vata imbalances, soothe the nervous system, and nourish the skin. For Vata types, **sesame oil** is ideal, while Pitta types may prefer **coconut oil** to cool the body. Abhyanga also improves circulation and reduces tension, making it a calming practice for women experiencing menopause.
- **Yoga and Pranayama**: Gentle yoga practices that focus on flexibility, balance, and grounding are beneficial for women during menopause. Specific poses such as **forward bends**, **restorative poses**, and **hip openers** help calm Vata and Pitta energies and ease stress. Pranayama techniques like **Nadi Shodhana** (alternate nostril breathing) and **Bhramari** (bee breath) help to reduce anxiety and promote emotional stability.
- **Meditation and Mindfulness**: Meditation can help ease emotional fluctuations, reduce stress, and improve mental clarity during menopause. Practices like mindfulness, loving-kindness meditation, or guided imagery can help women stay present and maintain emotional balance. By reducing mental chatter and promoting relaxation, these practices support mental well-being and help prevent feelings of overwhelm.

4. **Lifestyle Adjustments**

A balanced lifestyle is key to managing the changes that come with menopause. Ayurveda encourages women to maintain a consistent routine to help stabilize Vata and support overall health.

- **Sleep**: Adequate and restful sleep is vital during menopause. Ayurveda recommends a regular sleep schedule, with early bedtimes and a calming evening routine. Creating a peaceful, relaxing sleep environment, free from distractions, can help ease insomnia or night sweats.
- **Physical Activity**: Moderate exercise, such as walking, swimming, or yoga, helps to keep the body flexible, improve circulation, and reduce stress. It also supports digestion, energy levels, and overall vitality. Exercise is particularly beneficial for managing Kapha imbalances, such as weight gain and emotional stagnation.

Emotional and Spiritual Well-being

Ayurveda emphasizes that menopause is a spiritual as well as a physical transition. It is a time when women can embrace their inner wisdom, release past emotions, and focus on personal growth. Engaging in practices that promote emotional balance—such as journaling, creative expression, or spending time in nature—can support this transformative phase.

Ayurveda provides a comprehensive approach to managing the physical, emotional, and mental shifts that occur during menopause. By focusing on diet, herbal support, self-care, and lifestyle practices, Ayurveda helps women navigate this transition with grace, vitality, and balance. Rather than being a time of decline, menopause is viewed as an opportunity for empowerment and self-renewal. Through Ayurvedic principles, women can embrace this new phase of life and maintain health, happiness, and harmony.

Ayurveda for Men

In Ayurveda, men's health is approached holistically, focusing on maintaining balance between the body, mind, and spirit. The ancient system of medicine recognizes the unique needs of men and offers a comprehensive approach to achieving optimal health, vitality, and longevity. Ayurveda emphasizes the importance of balancing the doshas (Vata, Pitta, and Kapha), strengthening the digestive fire (Agni), and maintaining mental and emotional stability. This personalized and natural approach helps address common concerns for men such as energy levels, stress management, reproductive health, and overall well-being.

The Role of the Doshas in Men's Health

In Ayurveda, men's health is largely influenced by the balance of the three doshas, each of which governs specific aspects of the body and mind.

- **Vata** governs movement, the nervous system, and circulation. When Vata is out of balance, men may experience symptoms like anxiety, insomnia, fatigue, and joint issues. A Vata imbalance can lead to mental restlessness and physical dryness, affecting both physical and emotional well-being.
- **Pitta** is the dosha of heat, transformation, and metabolism. It governs digestion, metabolism, and energy. An imbalance in Pitta can manifest as irritability, inflammation, digestive disturbances, and conditions like acne or premature graying. Pitta imbalances are often linked to stress, anger, and burnout.
- **Kapha** governs structure, lubrication, and stability. It is associated with endurance and strength. When Kapha is out of balance, it can lead to weight gain, lethargy, and emotional stagnation. Kapha imbalances are often seen in men who experience emotional attachment, sluggishness, or difficulty in managing stress.

Ayurvedic Diet for Men's Health

In Ayurveda, food is considered medicine, and diet plays a crucial role in maintaining balance within the body. A personalized diet based on one's dosha and lifestyle can help manage energy levels, maintain a healthy weight, and promote overall vitality.

- **For Vata**: Men with a predominant Vata dosha benefit from warm, grounding, and nourishing foods. Foods like **whole grains**, **root vegetables**, and **warm soups** help soothe Vata's dryness and lightness. Adding healthy fats, such as **ghee**,

- **avocado**, and **nuts**, can help keep Vata in balance. Men with Vata imbalances should also avoid excessive caffeine and cold, raw foods, which can aggravate their dosha.
- **For Pitta**: To balance Pitta, men should opt for cooling, hydrating, and anti-inflammatory foods. **Leafy greens**, **cucumbers**, **coconut**, and **dairy** help reduce excess heat and support overall digestion. Pitta men should avoid spicy, sour, and oily foods, as these can cause inflammation, skin problems, and digestive disturbances.
- **For Kapha**: Men with a Kapha imbalance benefit from light, stimulating foods that promote circulation and energy. **Spices** like **ginger**, **turmeric**, and **black pepper** help stimulate digestion and prevent sluggishness. **Legumes, bitter greens**, and **leafy vegetables** support weight management and prevent excess Kapha buildup.

A balanced Ayurvedic diet encourages eating at regular intervals, avoiding overeating, and consuming easily digestible meals to support digestive health (Agni). **Triphala**, a blend of three fruits—**Amalaki, Bibhitaki**, and **Haritaki**—is commonly used to support digestion and detoxification.

Herbal Remedies for Men's Health

Ayurvedic herbs are powerful tools to promote energy, vitality, and address specific health concerns. Many herbs support hormonal balance, improve reproductive health, enhance stamina, and reduce stress.

- **Ashwagandha**: This adaptogenic herb is one of the most popular Ayurvedic remedies for men. It helps manage stress, improve mental clarity, and enhance physical strength. Ashwagandha is particularly beneficial for men experiencing fatigue, anxiety, or sexual dysfunction. It supports the adrenal glands and helps boost energy levels, making it ideal for men who experience stress-related imbalances.
- **Shilajit**: Known as a potent rejuvenator, Shilajit is used to enhance strength, stamina, and vitality. It is particularly effective in managing conditions like **low libido** or **erectile dysfunction** and supports overall reproductive health.
- **Gokshura** (Tribulus Terrestris): This herb is well known for its ability to improve sexual health, boost testosterone levels, and increase stamina. It is often used to address **low libido, infertility**, and **muscle weakness**.
- **Turmeric**: With its anti-inflammatory properties, turmeric is beneficial for reducing joint pain, skin conditions, and digestive issues. It also supports the liver and detoxification processes, enhancing overall health.
- **Brahmi**: Known for its ability to improve memory and cognitive function, Brahmi is also a great herb for reducing stress and anxiety. It promotes mental clarity and

emotional well-being, which is particularly important for men managing high levels of stress or anxiety.

Stress Management and Mental Health

Stress is one of the leading causes of health problems for men, affecting everything from cardiovascular health to digestive function and mental clarity. Ayurveda offers a variety of practices to help men manage stress, stay mentally focused, and promote emotional well-being.

1. **Pranayama (Breathing Exercises)**: **Nadi Shodhana** (alternate nostril breathing) and **Bhramari** (bee breath) are particularly effective for calming the nervous system, reducing anxiety, and improving mental clarity. Regular pranayama helps restore balance to Vata and Pitta energies and can reduce mental fatigue and stress.
2. **Meditation**: Ayurveda encourages daily meditation to reduce stress, improve focus, and promote emotional stability. Meditation practices help men disconnect from daily pressures, calm the mind, and foster a sense of peace and balance.
3. **Yoga**: Gentle yoga practices help improve flexibility, strengthen the body, and promote mental clarity. Poses like **Downward Dog**, **Child's Pose**, and **Mountain Pose** are ideal for reducing stress and promoting physical and emotional balance.
4. **Abhyanga (Self-Massage)**: Regular self-massage with warm oils can promote relaxation, improve circulation, and reduce tension. **Sesame oil** is particularly grounding for Vata types, while **coconut oil** is cooling for Pitta types. **Mustard oil** is stimulating and invigorating for Kapha types.

Maintaining Physical Health

In Ayurveda, maintaining good physical health involves not only a balanced diet and regular exercise but also ensuring that the body's internal energy flows freely.

- **Exercise**: Regular physical activity is essential for maintaining a healthy body and mind. Ayurveda recommends a balanced approach to exercise that involves both aerobic and strength-training exercises, depending on your dosha. Vata types benefit from grounding exercises like walking or swimming, while Pitta types can benefit from more challenging workouts like running or weightlifting. Kapha types should aim for vigorous exercise to stimulate circulation and prevent stagnation.
- **Sleep**: Adequate rest is essential for maintaining mental clarity, physical strength, and emotional stability. Ayurveda recommends going to bed early (before **10 PM**) and maintaining a consistent sleep schedule to help the body rejuvenate.

Sexual Health

In Ayurveda, sexual health is deeply connected to the balance of the doshas, the vitality of Agni (digestive fire), and emotional well-being. Erectile dysfunction, low libido, or premature ejaculation are common concerns for many men, especially as they age. Ayurvedic herbs like **Ashwagandha**, **Gokshura**, and **Shilajit** help promote sexual vitality, enhance libido, and address reproductive concerns.

Ayurveda also emphasizes the importance of a balanced lifestyle, which includes stress management, emotional well-being, and proper nutrition, all of which contribute to healthy sexual function.

Ayurveda offers a comprehensive and individualized approach to men's health that emphasizes balance, vitality, and overall well-being. By addressing the root causes of physical, emotional, and mental imbalances, Ayurveda supports men in achieving optimal health and longevity. Through a personalized approach that includes diet, herbs, exercise, and self-care practices, men can maintain strength, vitality, and mental clarity throughout their lives. Ayurveda's holistic methods empower men to embrace wellness with a natural and balanced lifestyle.

Ayurveda for Male Vitality

In Ayurveda, vitality is seen as a reflection of the balance between the body's physical energy, mental clarity, and emotional well-being. For men, maintaining vitality is crucial for overall health, as it affects everything from physical performance and energy levels to mental focus and emotional resilience. Ayurveda offers a comprehensive approach to enhancing male vitality by focusing on the balance of the doshas (Vata, Pitta, and Kapha), nourishing the body, and addressing lifestyle factors that may disrupt energy flow. By incorporating Ayurvedic principles, men can achieve sustained energy, improve stamina, and enjoy optimal physical, mental, and emotional health.

The Role of the Doshas in Male Vitality

In Ayurveda, vitality is closely linked to the balance of the three doshas, each of which influences different aspects of health:

- **Vata** governs movement, circulation, and nervous system function. When in balance, Vata provides energy, flexibility, and mental clarity. However, an imbalance in Vata, often due to stress, irregular sleep, or poor diet, can lead to fatigue, anxiety, and exhaustion. Vata is particularly prone to imbalances as men age, leading to decreased vitality and energy levels.
- **Pitta** controls digestion, metabolism, and heat. It is the dosha associated with transformation and energy. When Pitta is balanced, it supports strong digestion, physical endurance, and mental sharpness. However, excess Pitta can cause inflammation, irritability, and burnout, which diminishes vitality and can lead to fatigue, skin problems, and emotional instability.
- **Kapha** is responsible for structure, stability, and lubrication. While Kapha provides endurance and strength, an excess of Kapha can lead to sluggishness, weight gain, and lethargy, making it harder for men to maintain high energy levels. When Kapha is in balance, it supports stamina and a calm, grounded energy.

Maintaining vitality requires understanding how the doshas interact in the body and adjusting lifestyle, diet, and self-care practices to keep them in harmony.

Diet for Enhancing Vitality

Ayurveda emphasizes that food is the foundation of vitality. Proper digestion and nourishment support the body's energy reserves. A well-balanced diet that aligns with one's dosha can enhance vitality by improving digestion, metabolism, and nutrient absorption.

- **For Vata**: Grounding, warming foods help balance the dryness and irregularity that often accompany Vata imbalances. Foods like **whole grains**, **root vegetables**, **ghee**, and **nuts** provide warmth, nourishment, and moisture. Consuming **warm soups**, **stews**, and **cooked vegetables** helps stabilize energy and support digestion. Avoiding cold, dry, or raw foods is key to maintaining balance and preventing fatigue.
- **For Pitta**: Cooling foods help counteract the excess heat and intensity of Pitta. **Leafy greens**, **cucumbers**, **coconut**, and **dairy** products are excellent choices. Pitta types should avoid spicy, oily, and fried foods that can lead to inflammation and irritability. Foods that are both light and nourishing, such as **rice** and **pulses**, help support steady energy and maintain mental clarity.
- **For Kapha**: Light, stimulating foods help balance the heaviness and sluggishness of Kapha. **Spicy foods**, **legumes**, **bitter greens**, and **cruciferous vegetables** like broccoli and cauliflower boost metabolism and prevent energy stagnation. Avoiding overly rich or sweet foods, as well as minimizing dairy and fried items, helps prevent weight gain and promotes sustained energy.

Ayurvedic Herbs for Vitality

Ayurvedic herbs are powerful tools for boosting vitality and energy. Many herbs support hormonal balance, improve stamina, and enhance both physical and mental performance.

- **Ashwagandha**: Known as an adaptogen, **Ashwagandha** is one of the most renowned herbs for boosting male vitality. It helps the body adapt to stress, promotes physical strength, and enhances stamina. Ashwagandha is also beneficial for improving libido, enhancing sexual performance, and supporting muscle mass. It works by balancing Vata and Pitta and revitalizing the body's energy reserves.
- **Shilajit**: **Shilajit** is a potent mineral-rich substance used to enhance energy, stamina, and strength. It helps rejuvenate the body, increase endurance, and improve overall vitality. Shilajit also supports healthy testosterone levels and sexual health, making it an excellent choice for men looking to maintain vitality as they age.
- **Gokshura** (Tribulus Terrestris): This herb is widely used in Ayurveda to improve male reproductive health and vitality. It enhances libido, boosts testosterone levels, and increases energy. Gokshura is particularly beneficial for men with fatigue, low libido, or difficulty maintaining physical strength.

- **Brahmi:** Brahmi is a revered herb for mental clarity, cognitive function, and stress reduction. It improves focus, memory, and concentration, which contributes to mental vitality. Brahmi also has a calming effect, making it useful for managing anxiety or stress that can deplete energy.
- **Turmeric:** Known for its anti-inflammatory properties, **turmeric** supports joint health, reduces muscle soreness, and improves circulation. It helps maintain healthy blood flow and boosts energy levels by reducing inflammation in the body.

Lifestyle Practices to Boost Vitality

Along with diet and herbs, Ayurveda recommends lifestyle practices that enhance overall vitality and well-being. These practices focus on managing stress, improving physical strength, and supporting mental clarity.

- **Abhyanga (Self-Massage):** Regular self-massage with warm oils, such as **sesame oil** or **coconut oil**, is an Ayurvedic practice that supports vitality by improving circulation, reducing muscle tension, and calming the nervous system. Abhyanga promotes a sense of groundedness and replenishes energy, helping to maintain physical and mental balance.
- **Yoga and Pranayama:** **Yoga** is integral to enhancing physical and mental vitality. Regular practice improves flexibility, strengthens muscles, and boosts energy. Certain yoga poses, such as **Sun Salutations**, **Warrior Pose**, and **Downward Dog**, are particularly energizing and help promote vitality. **Pranayama** (breathing exercises) like **Nadi Shodhana** (alternate nostril breathing) and **Kapalbhati** (skull-shining breath) can help clear mental fog, reduce stress, and improve oxygen flow to the body.
- **Adequate Rest and Sleep:** Ayurveda emphasizes the importance of sleep for rejuvenating the body and restoring energy. Men should aim for **7-8 hours of restful sleep** each night, ideally going to bed early to align with the body's natural circadian rhythms. A consistent sleep routine helps regenerate physical strength, improve mental clarity, and maintain hormonal balance.
- **Exercise:** Regular physical activity is vital for maintaining vitality and energy. Ayurveda encourages a balanced approach to exercise, combining aerobic activity (like walking or swimming) with strength training to build stamina and maintain muscle mass. Men are advised to avoid overexertion, as it can deplete vital energy and lead to burnout.

Sexual Health and Vitality

Sexual vitality is an important aspect of male vitality in Ayurveda. Sexual health is linked to the balance of the doshas, and Ayurvedic herbs like **Ashwagandha**, **Shatavari**, and **Gokshura** are commonly used to support healthy libido, testosterone levels, and sexual function. A balanced diet, regular exercise, and stress management are essential for maintaining sexual health, and Ayurveda suggests practices such as **meditation** and **yoga** to reduce stress and improve overall vitality.

Ayurveda offers a personalized and holistic approach to enhancing male vitality by addressing physical, mental, and emotional health. By balancing the doshas, nourishing the body with the right foods and herbs, incorporating lifestyle practices such as yoga and pranayama, and managing stress, men can maintain sustained energy, physical strength, and mental clarity throughout their lives. Ayurveda provides the tools to support long-term vitality, ensuring that men feel strong, vibrant, and energized at every stage of life.

Ayurvedic Remedies for Common Men's Health Concerns

In Ayurveda, health is seen as the perfect balance between the mind, body, and spirit. For men, maintaining that balance is essential for overall well-being, as many common health concerns can be traced back to imbalances in the doshas (Vata, Pitta, and Kapha). Ayurveda offers natural remedies that address the root causes of these health issues, whether physical, mental, or emotional. By focusing on diet, lifestyle, and herbal support, Ayurvedic remedies can help men improve vitality, manage stress, and maintain health through the use of time-tested holistic approaches.

1. Stress and Anxiety Management

Stress is one of the most common health issues for men, affecting both mental and physical well-being. It can contribute to sleep disturbances, weight gain, high blood pressure, and emotional strain. Ayurveda believes that stress is primarily linked to imbalances in **Vata** and **Pitta** doshas.

- **Ashwagandha**: This adaptogenic herb is a cornerstone of Ayurvedic stress management. It helps reduce anxiety, improve mood, and promote emotional stability by balancing both **Vata** and **Pitta** energies. Ashwagandha also supports adrenal health, reduces the physical effects of stress, and enhances vitality.
- **Brahmi**: Known for its calming effects, **Brahmi** is particularly useful for Pitta-driven stress, which can lead to irritability, frustration, and mental burnout. This herb calms the nervous system, promotes mental clarity, and enhances cognitive function, making it ideal for managing anxiety and stress.
- **Meditation and Pranayama**: Regular **pranayama** (breathing exercises) like **Nadi Shodhana** (alternate nostril breathing) and **Bhramari** (bee breath) help calm the nervous system, reduce stress, and improve mental clarity. Meditation also plays a key role in grounding Vata energy, reducing mental restlessness, and fostering emotional well-being.

2. Low Energy and Fatigue

Fatigue is a common complaint for men, often linked to poor lifestyle choices, stress, or imbalances in digestion and metabolism. Ayurveda addresses low energy by focusing on digestive health, nutrition, and stress reduction.

- **Ginseng**: Known for its energizing properties, **Ginseng** enhances stamina, reduces fatigue, and improves physical endurance. It strengthens the **Kapha** dosha, which is associated with vitality and longevity.
- **Ashwagandha**: In addition to managing stress, **Ashwagandha** helps boost energy levels and combat fatigue. It is often used to enhance physical strength, improve sleep, and support the immune system.
- **Proper Nutrition**: Eating nourishing foods that support **Agni** (digestive fire) is crucial for maintaining energy levels. Warm, easily digestible foods such as **soups, stews, whole grains**, and **lentils** provide steady, long-lasting energy without burdening the digestive system.

3. Digestive Issues

Digestive problems such as bloating, indigestion, constipation, and acid reflux are common concerns for many men. Ayurveda stresses the importance of a strong digestive fire (Agni) for overall health and recommends dietary and herbal remedies to support digestion.

- **Triphala**: A blend of three fruits—**Amalaki, Bibhitaki,** and **Haritaki**—Triphala is a powerful herb that promotes healthy digestion, detoxifies the body, and supports regular bowel movements. It can be used to treat constipation and promote gut health.
- **Ginger**: **Ginger** is one of the most versatile Ayurvedic remedies for digestive issues. It stimulates **Agni**, improves circulation, and helps relieve symptoms of bloating, indigestion, and nausea. Drinking ginger tea after meals can aid digestion and reduce post-meal discomfort.
- **Fennel Seeds**: Fennel seeds are widely used in Ayurveda to support digestion. They are especially useful for men experiencing bloating or gas. Fennel helps relax the muscles of the gastrointestinal tract, improve digestion, and reduce bloating and cramping.
- **Cumin**: **Cumin** is a carminative herb, meaning it helps alleviate gas and bloating. It stimulates digestion, enhances nutrient absorption, and can be added to meals or consumed as a tea to improve digestive health.

4. Sexual Health and Libido

Maintaining sexual health is a significant concern for many men, particularly as they age. Low libido, erectile dysfunction, and reduced stamina are common issues that can stem from physical, emotional, or hormonal imbalances. Ayurveda offers numerous remedies to boost sexual health and vitality.

- **Shatavari**: Often used for women, **Shatavari** is also beneficial for men's reproductive health. It helps balance hormones, increase libido, and improve

sperm quality. It supports both physical stamina and emotional well-being, making it a great tonic for men seeking to enhance vitality.
- **Gokshura** (Tribulus Terrestris): **Gokshura** is known for its ability to increase testosterone levels and improve sexual function. It enhances libido, supports the prostate, and increases energy levels, making it a popular herb for treating erectile dysfunction and low libido.
- **Maca Root**: Maca is an adaptogen that boosts energy levels, stamina, and sexual health. It helps balance hormone levels and improves sexual desire and performance, particularly for men with stress-induced libido issues.
- **Shilajit**: A powerful rejuvenating herb, **Shilajit** is known for boosting testosterone, improving sexual stamina, and enhancing overall vitality. It increases energy levels, supports sexual health, and is particularly helpful for men experiencing fatigue or low libido.

5. Joint and Muscle Health

As men age, joint and muscle pain become more common due to wear and tear, inflammation, and poor circulation. Ayurveda promotes the use of anti-inflammatory herbs, regular exercise, and dietary changes to support joint and muscle health.

- **Turmeric**: **Turmeric** is a well-known anti-inflammatory herb used in Ayurveda to treat joint pain, muscle soreness, and conditions like arthritis. It helps reduce inflammation, improve circulation, and support overall joint health.
- **Ashwagandha**: In addition to its benefits for stress, **Ashwagandha** is also known for strengthening the muscles and improving flexibility. It supports joint health, reduces muscle stiffness, and enhances recovery after physical activity.
- **Ginger and Garlic**: Both **ginger** and **garlic** have anti-inflammatory properties and are frequently used in Ayurvedic treatments to relieve muscle pain and joint stiffness. They also improve circulation, which helps with the healing process.
- **Boswellia**: **Boswellia** (Indian frankincense) is another herb that has strong anti-inflammatory properties. It is used to treat conditions like osteoarthritis and joint pain, promoting mobility and comfort.

6. Mental Clarity and Cognitive Function

Mental sharpness, focus, and memory are essential components of overall vitality. Men who experience mental fatigue, brain fog, or emotional stress can benefit from Ayurvedic practices that enhance cognitive function and mental clarity.

- **Brahmi**: This herb is renowned for its ability to enhance memory, improve concentration, and calm the mind. It is particularly useful for men experiencing stress-related cognitive decline or mental fatigue.

- **Ashwagandha**: Besides its role in stress reduction, **Ashwagandha** also promotes mental clarity and enhances cognitive function. It improves memory, focus, and concentration by supporting the nervous system and reducing mental fatigue.
- **Ginkgo Biloba**: Known for improving blood circulation, particularly to the brain, **Ginkgo Biloba** supports memory function and mental clarity. It is often recommended for men who wish to maintain cognitive health as they age.

Ayurvedic remedies offer a natural, holistic approach to addressing common health concerns for men. By focusing on diet, herbs, and lifestyle practices, Ayurveda helps men improve energy levels, enhance sexual health, manage stress, support digestion, and maintain mental clarity. Through a personalized approach to health, Ayurveda promotes long-term vitality and well-being, helping men live healthier, more balanced lives.

Ayurveda and Beauty

In Ayurveda, beauty is not just about external appearance but is seen as the natural radiance that comes from within. The holistic system views beauty as a reflection of inner balance, where physical, emotional, and spiritual well-being all play a part in how we express ourselves on the outside. Ayurvedic beauty practices focus on nourishing the body, mind, and soul to bring out a healthy, glowing complexion, lustrous hair, and overall vitality. Ayurveda encourages a personalized approach to beauty, taking into account the individual's dosha (Vata, Pitta, Kapha), lifestyle, diet, and emotional state to restore balance and enhance natural beauty.

Ayurvedic Principles of Beauty

The Ayurvedic concept of beauty is rooted in the balance of the **doshas**, which govern different aspects of the body and mind. When the doshas are in harmony, the body's natural radiance shines through. However, imbalances in these energies can lead to common beauty concerns such as dull skin, hair loss, acne, or premature aging. Ayurveda offers specific remedies based on an individual's doshic constitution to restore equilibrium and support healthy skin, hair, and overall appearance.

- **Vata** types tend to have dry, sensitive skin that can be prone to premature aging, fine lines, and dryness. They benefit from moisturizing, nourishing treatments that balance their dryness and restore hydration.
- **Pitta** types often have sensitive skin prone to acne, rosacea, or inflammation. Cooling and soothing treatments help reduce redness, irritation, and inflammation.
- **Kapha** types typically have oily, thicker skin but may also struggle with congestion, acne, or dullness. Balancing Kapha requires stimulating treatments that prevent stagnation and enhance circulation.

Diet and Nutrition for Radiant Skin

In Ayurveda, food is considered the foundation of beauty, and what you consume plays a significant role in your complexion. A diet that balances the doshas can promote healthy skin and enhance natural beauty.

- **For Vata**: Foods that are moist, grounding, and nourishing are essential for Vata types. Warm soups, stews, and healthy fats like **ghee**, **avocados**, and **nuts** hydrate

dry skin and promote a glowing complexion. Vata types should also avoid excessive caffeine, alcohol, and raw foods, as they can further dry out the skin.
- **For Pitta**: Cooling, hydrating, and anti-inflammatory foods are key for Pitta types. **Cucumbers**, **coconut**, **leafy greens**, and **dairy** help soothe inflamed or irritated skin. Foods like **mint**, **melons**, and **rice** help calm Pitta heat and reduce redness, acne, or rosacea. Pitta types should avoid spicy, greasy foods and excessive caffeine or alcohol, which can exacerbate inflammation.
- **For Kapha**: Light, stimulating foods that promote digestion and circulation are important for Kapha types. **Bitter greens**, **legumes**, and **spices** like **turmeric**, **ginger**, and **black pepper** help detoxify and prevent congestion in the skin. Kapha types should avoid heavy, oily, or sugary foods that may contribute to acne or dullness.

Drinking plenty of water and herbal teas such as **chamomile** or **ginger** helps detoxify the body, hydrate the skin, and flush out impurities.

Ayurvedic Skincare

Ayurveda offers a wide range of natural remedies for skincare, focusing on balancing the doshas, supporting digestion, and detoxifying the body. Ayurvedic beauty rituals typically involve using natural oils, herbs, and massage techniques to promote healthy, glowing skin.

- **Abhyanga (Self-Massage)**: Daily self-massage with warm oils is one of the most effective Ayurvedic practices for nourishing the skin. **Sesame oil** is ideal for Vata types, providing warmth and moisture to dry skin, while **coconut oil** is cooling and soothing for Pitta types. **Mustard oil** is stimulating and detoxifying for Kapha types. Abhyanga promotes circulation, helps eliminate toxins (Ama), and leaves the skin soft, glowing, and rejuvenated.
- **Herbal Face Masks**: Ayurveda uses a variety of herbs and ingredients to create nourishing face masks that target different skin concerns. A simple **turmeric** and **milk** mask can brighten the skin and reduce inflammation, while a mixture of **gram flour** and **turmeric** acts as a natural exfoliant to cleanse and purify the skin. **Aloe vera**, **sandalwood**, and **neem** are other herbs that help soothe, cool, and reduce redness or acne.
- **Rose Water**: Known for its cooling and soothing properties, **rose water** is often used to tone the skin and reduce irritation. It helps maintain a balanced pH, hydrate the skin, and reduce redness, making it ideal for Pitta types with sensitive or inflamed skin.
- **Neem Oil**: Neem is revered in Ayurveda for its purifying properties. **Neem oil** can be used to treat acne, reduce skin irritation, and promote clear skin. It has natural antibacterial and antifungal properties that make it ideal for oily or acne-prone skin.

- **Kumkumadi Oil**: Kumkumadi oil is a luxurious Ayurvedic beauty oil known for its ability to brighten and rejuvenate the skin. A blend of saffron, sandalwood, and other herbs, it helps reduce pigmentation, improve complexion, and nourish dry or aging skin.

Ayurvedic Hair Care

Hair health in Ayurveda is deeply connected to the balance of the doshas. Hair problems such as thinning, dryness, dandruff, or premature graying can be alleviated through dietary changes, herbal remedies, and regular hair care practices.

- **Amla**: This powerhouse herb is rich in vitamin C and antioxidants, making it a staple in Ayurvedic hair care. **Amla** nourishes the scalp, strengthens hair follicles, and prevents premature graying. It is often used in hair oils or taken internally to promote healthy, shiny hair.
- **Bhringraj**: Known as the "king of herbs" for hair health, **Bhringraj** helps stimulate hair growth, prevent hair loss, and improve the overall texture of the hair. It can be used in hair oils or as a hair mask to restore health and shine to the hair.
- **Shikakai**: **Shikakai** is a natural cleanser that gently cleans the scalp and hair without stripping away natural oils. It is often used in hair powders and oils to promote healthy hair growth, improve shine, and reduce dandruff.
- **Coconut Oil**: **Coconut oil** is an excellent conditioner for the hair, providing deep hydration and nourishment. It helps prevent dryness, reduces frizz, and promotes healthy, strong hair.

The Role of Lifestyle in Ayurvedic Beauty

In Ayurveda, beauty is not just about external treatments but about overall lifestyle and self-care. Maintaining a balanced routine that supports physical health, mental clarity, and emotional well-being is key to achieving lasting beauty.

- **Sleep**: Adequate and restful sleep is vital for rejuvenating the skin and promoting natural beauty. Ayurveda recommends going to bed early and waking up early to maintain the body's natural circadian rhythms. Proper rest allows the body to repair itself and rejuvenate cells, leading to clearer, more radiant skin.
- **Exercise**: Regular exercise promotes healthy circulation, reduces stress, and helps detoxify the body, which in turn supports glowing skin. Ayurveda recommends moderate exercise that aligns with your doshic constitution.
- **Mindfulness**: Mental and emotional well-being are crucial for beauty in Ayurveda. Practices like meditation, yoga, and deep breathing exercises help reduce stress, improve sleep, and promote an inner calm that radiates on the outside.

Ayurvedic beauty is rooted in the belief that true beauty comes from balance, vitality, and self-care. By nourishing the body from within with the right foods, herbs, and lifestyle practices, and by using natural skincare and hair care remedies, Ayurveda helps individuals enhance their natural radiance. Whether through specific treatments for skin or hair or holistic lifestyle changes that promote inner balance, Ayurveda offers a timeless approach to beauty that celebrates individuality and supports long-lasting well-being.

Ayurvedic Skin Care

In Ayurveda, the health of the skin is viewed as a reflection of the balance within the body, mind, and spirit. According to this ancient system of healing, the skin's condition is influenced by the balance of the **doshas** (Vata, Pitta, and Kapha), digestion (Agni), and the presence of toxins (Ama). Healthy, radiant skin is achieved when the internal systems are in harmony, and Ayurveda offers a holistic approach to skincare that addresses not just the external skin but also the internal factors that influence it. Through personalized diet, herbal remedies, lifestyle practices, and self-care rituals, Ayurveda helps support a clear, youthful complexion and maintains skin health.

Ayurvedic Approach to Skin Health

Ayurveda identifies that skin problems often arise due to an imbalance in the doshas. Each dosha affects the skin differently, and understanding your dosha type can help tailor skincare routines that restore balance and promote radiant skin.

- **Vata**: Vata types generally have dry, thin, and sensitive skin. Imbalances in Vata can lead to dryness, wrinkles, and premature aging. To balance Vata, Ayurveda recommends moisturizing treatments, hydration, and nourishment to combat skin dryness.
- **Pitta**: Pitta types typically have oily, sensitive skin that is prone to redness, acne, or inflammation. When Pitta is imbalanced, it can lead to conditions like acne, rosacea, or sunburn. Cooling and soothing treatments, as well as anti-inflammatory herbs, are ideal for Pitta skin.
- **Kapha**: Kapha types tend to have thicker, oilier skin that can be prone to acne, blackheads, and congestion. When out of balance, Kapha can cause the skin to feel heavy, congested, or dull. For Kapha skin, Ayurvedic treatments focus on cleansing, detoxifying, and improving circulation.

Ayurvedic Skincare Rituals

Daily self-care rituals are central to Ayurvedic skincare. Ayurveda believes that beauty comes from within and that the external skin reflects the inner balance. Regular cleansing, moisturizing, and nourishing rituals, using natural oils and herbs, are essential for maintaining healthy skin.

1. **Cleansing**:
    Ayurveda encourages the use of natural cleansers that maintain the skin's balance without stripping it of its natural oils. **Gram flour** (Chickpea flour) is a popular Ayurvedic cleanser that gently exfoliates and cleanses the skin. **Honey**, with its antibacterial properties, is often used as a cleanser for its ability to purify and hydrate the skin.
    - **Vata types** should use mild, moisturizing cleansers like **milk** or **rose water** to maintain hydration.
    - **Pitta types** benefit from cooling and soothing cleansers such as **coconut milk** or **aloe vera** to calm irritated or inflamed skin.
    - **Kapha types** can use deeper cleansing agents like **turmeric** or **neem**, which help clear excess oil and promote clear, fresh skin.
2. **Exfoliation**:
    Exfoliation is essential for removing dead skin cells, improving circulation, and promoting healthy cell regeneration. Ayurvedic exfoliants typically use natural ingredients like **sandalwood powder, rice flour,** or **turmeric** to exfoliate the skin gently.
    - **Vata types** can benefit from mild exfoliation using **milk and honey** to nourish and hydrate dry skin.
    - **Pitta types** should opt for cooling, gentle exfoliants like **rose powder** and **sandalwood** that soothe inflammation.
    - **Kapha types** may use more stimulating exfoliants, like **ground almonds** or **turmeric**, which help clear pores and balance oil production.
3. **Moisturizing**:
    Ayurveda emphasizes the importance of moisturizing to nourish the skin and prevent dryness. Depending on your dosha, the right oils and creams can replenish the skin's moisture balance.
    - **Vata types** benefit from **sesame oil** or **almond oil**, which are rich in fatty acids and help lock in moisture.
    - **Pitta types** can use **coconut oil** or **rose oil**, both of which cool and soothe the skin while providing hydration.
    - **Kapha types** may prefer lighter oils, such as **grapeseed oil** or **sunflower oil**, which provide hydration without making the skin feel greasy.
4. **Face Masks**:
    Ayurvedic face masks use natural ingredients that target specific skin concerns. These masks often contain ingredients like **turmeric, sandalwood, neem,** and **aloe vera**, known for their healing and purifying properties.
    - **Vata types** can use masks made with **honey and avocado** to hydrate and nourish dry skin.
    - **Pitta types** benefit from cooling masks made with **cucumber, rose water,** or **sandalwood**, which calm redness and irritation.
    - **Kapha types** can use masks with **turmeric, neem,** or **fuller's earth** to detoxify and control oiliness, promoting clear, balanced skin.

5. **Herbal Oils and Balms**:
   Ayurvedic oils are often infused with herbs that have healing, anti-inflammatory, and rejuvenating properties. Regular use of these oils helps nourish the skin deeply, improve elasticity, and combat signs of aging.
   - **Vata types** should use oils such as **sandalwood oil**, **lavender oil**, or **rose oil**, which are deeply moisturizing and soothing.
   - **Pitta types** benefit from **aloe vera gel**, **coconut oil**, or **turmeric oil**, which help cool and calm the skin.
   - **Kapha types** can use oils like **tea tree oil** or **neem oil**, known for their purifying properties, to control acne and oily skin.

Ayurvedic Herbs for Skin Health

Herbs are an essential part of Ayurvedic skincare, as they can address various skin conditions and support overall health. Some common Ayurvedic herbs for skincare include:

- **Turmeric**: Known for its anti-inflammatory and antibacterial properties, turmeric is a powerful herb for healing acne, reducing redness, and brightening the complexion. It also helps combat premature aging by promoting collagen production.
- **Neem**: **Neem** is used for its purifying and antibacterial properties, making it ideal for treating acne, eczema, and other skin infections. It helps detoxify the skin and prevent breakouts.
- **Aloe Vera**: **Aloe vera** is a cooling herb that soothes irritated skin, reduces redness, and promotes hydration. It is particularly effective for calming sunburn or inflammation.
- **Sandalwood**: **Sandalwood** has cooling and calming properties, making it effective for reducing inflammation and redness. It is used in Ayurvedic masks, creams, and oils for its skin-soothing benefits.
- **Rose**: **Rose** is known for its cooling, anti-inflammatory properties. It helps balance moisture levels, tone the skin, and calm irritation. **Rose water** is also commonly used as a toner to refresh and hydrate the skin.

Ayurveda and Skin Aging

In Ayurveda, the approach to aging is centered around balance and maintaining the health of **Ojas**, the vital energy that sustains life. When Ojas is strong, it supports radiant, youthful skin and protects against the effects of aging.

- **Amalaki (Indian Gooseberry)**: Rich in vitamin C and antioxidants, **Amalaki** is an essential herb for fighting premature aging. It strengthens the immune system, supports collagen production, and helps maintain the skin's youthful elasticity.

- **Ghee**: **Ghee** is a rejuvenating food that helps nourish the skin from the inside out. It hydrates dry skin, promotes elasticity, and reduces the appearance of fine lines and wrinkles.
- **Yoga and Pranayama**: Regular **yoga** and **pranayama** (breathing exercises) enhance circulation, detoxify the body, and reduce stress, which helps prevent the signs of aging. These practices promote the natural glow of the skin by encouraging internal balance and vitality.

Ayurvedic skincare is not just about external beauty but about creating harmony between the body and mind. By addressing the root causes of skin imbalances and using natural ingredients tailored to your dosha, Ayurveda helps promote healthy, glowing skin. Regular self-care rituals, combined with the right diet, herbs, and lifestyle practices, allow individuals to achieve radiant skin while maintaining long-term health and balance. Ayurveda encourages a holistic approach to beauty, where true radiance comes from within, and external treatments simply enhance this natural glow.

Natural Hair Care in Ayurveda

In Ayurveda, healthy hair is seen as a reflection of overall well-being, with both internal and external factors influencing its condition. The ancient system views hair health as closely tied to the balance of the **doshas** (Vata, Pitta, and Kapha), **Agni** (digestive fire), and the elimination of **Ama** (toxins). Ayurvedic hair care is not just about using topical treatments but emphasizes a holistic approach that includes diet, lifestyle, stress management, and the use of natural, herb-based remedies to nourish and maintain healthy, vibrant hair.

Ayurvedic Principles for Healthy Hair

In Ayurveda, hair is considered a byproduct of the body's tissues, known as **Rasa** (the lymphatic fluid), which is nourished by food and digestion. The health of Rasa depends on proper digestion (**Agni**) and the balance of the doshas. Each dosha affects the hair in unique ways, and understanding this connection is crucial for creating an effective hair care routine.

- **Vata**: Vata types tend to have dry, brittle, and thinning hair. An imbalance in Vata can lead to hair loss, dandruff, and frizz. Balancing Vata requires nourishment and hydration to prevent dryness and improve the hair's strength.
- **Pitta**: Pitta governs heat, metabolism, and transformation. When Pitta is out of balance, it can lead to hair thinning, premature graying, and scalp irritation. Cooling treatments that calm the scalp and reduce inflammation are key for Pitta types.
- **Kapha**: Kapha types usually have thick, strong hair but can experience excess oil, dandruff, or scalp congestion if Kapha becomes imbalanced. Stimulating and detoxifying treatments are ideal for keeping Kapha in check.

Ayurvedic Hair Care Routine

A balanced Ayurvedic hair care routine incorporates cleansing, nourishing, and strengthening the hair and scalp while considering one's doshic constitution and any imbalances.

1. **Oils for Hair Nourishment**

In Ayurveda, oils play a critical role in hair health. They nourish the hair, calm the scalp, and promote growth by strengthening hair roots and improving circulation.

- **For Vata: Sesame oil** is ideal for Vata types as it provides deep nourishment, reduces dryness, and strengthens hair follicles. It also improves circulation to the scalp, supporting healthy hair growth.
- **For Pitta: Coconut oil** is cooling and soothing, making it an excellent choice for Pitta types who may suffer from scalp irritation or inflammation. It hydrates the scalp, balances excess heat, and prevents premature graying.
- **For Kapha: Mustard oil** is invigorating and stimulating, ideal for Kapha types who need help with circulation and detoxification. It helps to clear excess oil from the scalp and keeps the hair follicles clean, reducing dandruff.

Massaging the scalp with warm oil regularly promotes relaxation, reduces stress, improves circulation, and stimulates hair growth. The Ayurvedic practice of **Abhyanga** (self-massage) is an excellent way to promote hair health, improve circulation, and nourish the hair from root to tip.

2. **Herbal Hair Masks and Treatments**

Ayurvedic herbs offer natural, potent solutions for hair care, addressing issues like dandruff, hair thinning, premature graying, and scalp irritation. These herbs provide nourishment and healing properties without harsh chemicals.

- **Brahmi**: Known for its ability to strengthen hair and improve mental clarity, **Brahmi** is one of the most widely used herbs for promoting hair growth. It is often used in oils or as part of a hair mask to improve circulation and nourish the hair follicles.
- **Amla** (Indian Gooseberry): Rich in vitamin C and antioxidants, **Amla** is known for its ability to promote hair growth, prevent hair loss, and reduce premature graying. It strengthens hair, improves its texture, and prevents damage from environmental stressors.
- **Fenugreek**: **Fenugreek** seeds are rich in proteins and nicotinic acid, which help stimulate hair growth, strengthen hair shafts, and prevent hair loss. A fenugreek paste or oil treatment can help condition the hair and prevent dandruff.
- **Hibiscus**: **Hibiscus** flowers are often used to create a nourishing hair mask that promotes hair growth, prevents hair loss, and adds natural shine. The plant's high vitamin C content also helps prevent scalp infections.
- **Neem**: Known for its antibacterial and antifungal properties, **Neem** helps cleanse the scalp, reduce dandruff, and improve overall hair health. Neem oil or a paste made from crushed neem leaves can be massaged into the scalp to prevent scalp conditions like itching or irritation.

Ayurvedic Herbs for Scalp Health

Healthy hair begins with a healthy scalp. In Ayurveda, a clean, nourished, and well-balanced scalp is essential for optimal hair growth. Several herbs are used to address common scalp concerns such as dandruff, irritation, and oil buildup.

- **Neem**: As mentioned, **Neem** is ideal for maintaining scalp health. Its antifungal properties help combat dandruff and scalp infections, keeping the scalp clean and free from excess oil and buildup.
- **Aloe Vera**: **Aloe vera** soothes an inflamed or irritated scalp, reducing itching and redness. It has hydrating properties that help balance the scalp's moisture levels and prevent dryness or excess oil.
- **Tea Tree Oil**: **Tea tree oil** is a powerful antiseptic and is commonly used to treat dandruff, fungal infections, and itchy scalps. It clears clogged hair follicles and promotes healthy hair growth.

Diet for Healthy Hair

In Ayurveda, diet plays an essential role in maintaining healthy hair. A well-balanced diet that supports **Agni** (digestive fire) helps the body absorb nutrients efficiently and promotes strong, lustrous hair. Ayurveda emphasizes the consumption of nutrient-rich foods that nourish both the body and hair.

- **Vata** types should consume grounding foods like **sweet potatoes**, **avocados**, **almonds**, and **ghee** to nourish their dry hair and skin. Warm, cooked meals are preferred, as they support digestion and enhance the absorption of nutrients.
- **Pitta** types should incorporate cooling foods like **coconut**, **cucumbers**, **leafy greens**, and **dairy** into their diet to soothe inflammation and prevent heat-related scalp issues like redness or premature graying.
- **Kapha** types benefit from light, stimulating foods like **bitter greens**, **spices** such as **ginger** and **black pepper**, and **legumes** to promote circulation and prevent excess oil buildup in the scalp.

Additionally, ensuring adequate hydration is key. Drinking **herbal teas** such as **chamomile**, **ginger**, and **mint** can improve circulation, reduce stress, and support digestion, all of which contribute to healthier hair.

Lifestyle Practices to Enhance Hair Health

In addition to diet and topical treatments, Ayurvedic lifestyle practices play a significant role in promoting healthy hair.

- **Regular Exercise**: Regular physical activity promotes circulation and ensures that essential nutrients reach the hair follicles, helping stimulate hair growth.

- **Sleep**: Ayurveda stresses the importance of getting adequate, restful sleep for overall health, including hair health. Sleep supports the body's natural detoxification and rejuvenation processes, helping to maintain a healthy scalp and hair.
- **Stress Management**: Chronic stress can lead to hair loss and thinning, as it disrupts the balance of the doshas and affects digestion. Ayurveda recommends practices like yoga, meditation, and deep breathing exercises to manage stress and restore balance.

Ayurvedic hair care is a comprehensive approach that nurtures the hair and scalp from the inside out. By focusing on the balance of the doshas, nourishing the body with a balanced diet, and using natural herbs and oils, Ayurveda provides a holistic solution for maintaining healthy, vibrant hair. Whether you are dealing with dry, thinning hair, dandruff, or scalp irritation, Ayurvedic treatments offer gentle, effective remedies to promote hair growth, improve texture, and restore balance to the scalp, ensuring that your hair reflects both internal health and external beauty.

Ayurvedic Oral Care

In Ayurveda, oral health is considered an integral part of overall well-being, deeply connected to the balance of the doshas and the body's internal systems. Ayurveda believes that the mouth is a gateway to the body and a reflection of a person's digestive fire (**Agni**), which directly influences the health of the teeth, gums, and tongue. Oral hygiene practices are not just about cleaning the teeth but are seen as a holistic approach to detoxifying the body, balancing the doshas, and promoting overall health. By incorporating natural remedies, diet, and lifestyle practices, Ayurvedic oral care supports the health of the mouth while also benefiting the entire system.

Ayurvedic Principles of Oral Care

Oral health, according to Ayurveda, is not merely cosmetic but serves as an important indicator of internal balance. When the digestive system is healthy, the mouth is also healthy. However, imbalances in **Agni** (digestive fire), **Ama** (toxins), or the doshas can lead to oral health issues like bad breath, tooth decay, gum disease, and mouth ulcers. Ayurveda emphasizes the importance of both **external hygiene** and **internal balance**, which is achieved through proper diet, detoxification, and oral care routines.

Ayurvedic Practices for Oral Hygiene

1. **Oil Pulling (Kavala or Gandusha)**

One of the most well-known Ayurvedic practices for oral health is **oil pulling**, or **Kavala**, a technique that involves swishing oil in the mouth to cleanse the teeth, gums, and tongue. This practice is believed to detoxify the mouth and remove **Ama** (toxins), which can lead to oral diseases and bad breath.

- **Sesame oil** is commonly recommended for oil pulling due to its warming properties and ability to balance Vata and Kapha doshas.
- **Coconut oil**, with its cooling properties, is also commonly used, especially for Pitta imbalances, as it helps soothe inflamed gums and freshens the breath.

To practice oil pulling, take a tablespoon of oil and swish it in your mouth for 10–20 minutes. Avoid swallowing the oil, as it contains toxins and bacteria that have been pulled from the mouth. Afterward, spit the oil out and rinse your mouth with warm water.

2. Tongue Scraping

Tongue scraping is an essential part of Ayurvedic oral care. Ayurveda suggests that the tongue is a direct reflection of the health of the digestive system, and toxins (Ama) often accumulate on the tongue. Scraping the tongue regularly helps remove this coating and promotes better digestion and fresh breath.

Using a **copper** or **stainless steel** tongue scraper, gently scrape from the back of the tongue to the front. This should be done each morning before brushing the teeth to eliminate toxins and improve oral hygiene.

3. Herbal Mouth Rinses

Ayurvedic herbs offer natural antibacterial and anti-inflammatory properties that support healthy gums, teeth, and fresh breath. Regular use of herbal mouth rinses helps cleanse the mouth, prevent gum disease, and soothe irritation.

- **Neem**: Known for its antibacterial and antifungal properties, **neem** is often used in Ayurvedic oral care to prevent gum disease, fight bad breath, and protect against plaque buildup. **Neem** mouthwashes or **neem-based toothpaste** can help maintain healthy gums and prevent infections.
- **Triphala**: A combination of **Amalaki**, **Bibhitaki**, and **Haritaki**, **Triphala** is known for its detoxifying and rejuvenating properties. It is used to rinse the mouth to reduce inflammation, fight bacteria, and promote oral health.
- **Clove**: **Clove oil** is commonly used for its antiseptic and pain-relieving properties. It can help manage toothaches, prevent bad breath, and reduce gum inflammation.

To make an Ayurvedic mouth rinse, you can steep herbs like **neem** or **clove** in water, strain, and use it as a mouthwash for maintaining oral health.

4. Ayurvedic Toothpowder and Pastes

Traditional Ayurvedic toothpastes and powders are made with natural ingredients that clean the teeth, prevent decay, and promote healthy gums. These remedies are often free from harmful chemicals, fluoride, and synthetic additives, making them gentle and effective.

- **Baking soda** or **powdered charcoal** mixed with herbs like **neem**, **clove**, and **turmeric** can be used to clean teeth effectively. **Turmeric** helps with inflammation and can also whiten teeth naturally.
- **Neem**: Neem is one of the most powerful Ayurvedic herbs for dental care due to its antibacterial properties. Neem-based toothpastes or powders can prevent tooth decay, fight bacteria, and promote overall oral hygiene.

- **Miswak**: The **Miswak tree** has long been used in Ayurveda for dental care. The bark and twigs of the Miswak are naturally antiseptic and can be chewed to clean the teeth and gums. It helps remove plaque, fight bacteria, and freshen breath.

To make a simple Ayurvedic tooth powder, mix **neem powder, baking soda, clove powder**, and **turmeric**. This powder can be used with a wet toothbrush to clean the teeth.

5. **Diet and Oral Health**

Ayurveda emphasizes that the state of the digestive system directly impacts oral health. A balanced diet supports not just digestion but also the health of teeth and gums. According to Ayurveda, the following dietary practices promote healthy teeth and gums:

- **Consume cooling foods** like cucumbers, melons, and leafy greens to reduce inflammation and heat in the mouth, particularly for those with **Pitta** imbalances.
- **Avoid overly spicy, acidic, and sugary foods** that can irritate the gums, promote plaque buildup, and lead to tooth decay.
- **Eat fiber-rich foods** such as apples, carrots, and celery, which help stimulate the production of saliva, cleanse the teeth naturally, and reduce the buildup of plaque.
- **Hydrate well** by drinking warm water throughout the day to support healthy digestion and oral health.

6. **Stress Management and Oral Health**

In Ayurveda, stress is seen as a major contributor to oral health problems. Stress can cause **Vata imbalances**, leading to conditions like teeth grinding (**bruxism**), gum disease, and dry mouth. Incorporating stress-relieving practices into your daily routine can support both your mental and oral health.

- **Meditation** and **pranayama** (breathing exercises) help calm the nervous system, reduce stress, and promote overall balance, which directly benefits oral health.
- **Yoga** helps release tension in the jaw and mouth, preventing conditions like teeth grinding and temporomandibular joint (TMJ) disorders.

Ayurvedic Remedies for Specific Oral Health Concerns

1. **Bad Breath (Halitosis)**:
   Bad breath in Ayurveda is often associated with **Ama** (toxins) and digestive issues. Oil pulling with **sesame oil** or **coconut oil** and herbal mouth rinses with **neem** or **mint** can help eliminate bacteria and freshen the breath.
2. **Tooth Decay**:
   To prevent tooth decay, Ayurveda recommends oil pulling, the use of **neem** toothpaste, and the regular practice of **tongue scraping**. Additionally, a diet rich

in calcium, such as **sesame seeds**, **almonds**, and **leafy greens**, helps maintain strong teeth.
3. **Gum Disease (Gingivitis)**:
   For gum inflammation, herbal rinses made from **turmeric** or **clove** can help reduce swelling and fight bacteria. Regular **oil pulling** with **neem oil** helps maintain healthy gums and prevent infections.

Ayurvedic oral care offers a natural and holistic approach to maintaining a healthy mouth. By addressing the root causes of oral health issues through diet, lifestyle, and herbal treatments, Ayurveda promotes not only a clean mouth but also a balanced, toxin-free body. With regular practice of oil pulling, tongue scraping, and using herbal mouth rinses or tooth powders, one can enjoy long-term oral health that extends beyond just the teeth and gums. By focusing on both the internal and external factors, Ayurvedic oral care helps ensure that your mouth remains healthy, clean, and free from disease.

Ayurveda and Aging

In Ayurveda, aging is viewed as a natural and inevitable part of life, where the body's vital energy gradually diminishes over time. Rather than seeing aging as a decline, Ayurveda approaches it as a process of transformation, encouraging individuals to age gracefully with vitality, health, and balance. The key to maintaining youthful vigor and wellness lies in harmonizing the **doshas** (Vata, Pitta, and Kapha), strengthening **Ojas** (the body's vital essence), and supporting **Agni** (digestive fire). Through proper lifestyle, diet, herbs, and rejuvenation practices, Ayurveda offers effective tools for mitigating the effects of aging, promoting longevity, and preserving vitality throughout life.

The Role of Doshas in Aging

Each dosha plays a significant role in the aging process, influencing how we age and what health issues we may experience in later years. Ayurveda believes that when the doshas are in balance, the aging process is gradual and healthy. Imbalances, on the other hand, accelerate aging and may lead to disease.

- **Vata**: Vata governs movement and is associated with qualities such as dryness, coldness, and irregularity. As we age, Vata tends to increase, leading to symptoms like dry skin, brittle bones, and mental confusion. **Vata imbalance** can also cause issues like joint pain, memory loss, and digestive irregularities. Vata's tendency toward dryness makes it essential for aging individuals to focus on hydration, nourishment, and grounding practices to prevent the quickening of aging symptoms.
- **Pitta**: Pitta governs transformation, metabolism, and heat. As we grow older, an excess of Pitta can cause premature graying, thinning hair, skin rashes, or digestive issues. **Pitta imbalances** can lead to conditions related to inflammation, such as arthritis or hypertension. Cooling, soothing practices and avoiding excess heat are critical for aging individuals with a Pitta constitution to maintain balance and prevent rapid aging.
- **Kapha**: Kapha governs stability, structure, and lubrication. As we age, **Kapha imbalances** may manifest as weight gain, sluggishness, or emotional stagnation. The key to aging gracefully with Kapha is to keep the metabolism active, avoid excess weight gain, and stimulate circulation through regular physical activity and a stimulating diet.

Rejuvenation in Ayurveda (Rasayana Therapy)

Ayurveda's approach to slowing the aging process focuses on **Rasayana** therapy, a set of practices that promote rejuvenation, strengthen the immune system, and increase **Ojas** (vital energy). Rasayana enhances longevity by improving the health of tissues, promoting mental clarity, and slowing down the degeneration of the body.

- **Herbal Rasayanas**: Herbs such as **Ashwagandha**, **Amalaki**, **Shatavari**, and **Brahmi** are frequently used in Rasayana therapy. **Amalaki**, rich in vitamin C and antioxidants, is one of the most potent rejuvenating herbs for anti-aging. It promotes skin health, improves digestion, and strengthens the immune system.
- **Turmeric**: **Turmeric** is another key herb known for its anti-inflammatory and antioxidant properties. It helps protect the skin, fight oxidative stress, and reduce the signs of aging. **Turmeric** enhances **Agni** and **Ojas**, promoting overall vitality and slowing down the degenerative effects of aging.
- **Ghee**: Ghee, or clarified butter, is considered one of the most important Rasayana foods in Ayurveda. It nourishes the tissues, enhances digestion, and supports the nervous system. **Ghee** is believed to promote longevity and vitality when used in moderation, especially for those with Vata imbalances.

Diet for Healthy Aging

Ayurveda places great emphasis on the importance of diet in maintaining balance and preventing premature aging. A diet that supports digestion, strengthens **Ojas**, and balances the doshas is essential for slowing the aging process.

- **For Vata**: Aging individuals with a predominance of Vata benefit from warm, moist, and grounding foods. Soups, stews, and **whole grains** like **rice**, **quinoa**, and **oats** are nourishing and help prevent dryness and irregularity. Healthy fats, such as **avocado**, **ghee**, and **nuts**, provide essential nourishment to dry skin and tissues. Avoiding cold, raw foods and excessive caffeine can help maintain balance and prevent Vata-related aging issues.
- **For Pitta**: Pitta types should focus on cooling, anti-inflammatory foods to prevent excess heat, which can accelerate aging. **Leafy greens**, **cucumbers**, **coconut**, and **dairy** are ideal for soothing Pitta and reducing inflammation. Reducing spicy, sour, and oily foods, as well as alcohol, helps maintain balance and preserve youthful skin and energy levels.
- **For Kapha**: For Kapha types, a stimulating and light diet is recommended to avoid sluggishness and weight gain. Foods like **bitter greens**, **legumes**, and **spices** like **ginger**, **black pepper**, and **turmeric** help increase circulation, improve digestion, and stimulate metabolism. Avoiding heavy, greasy, and sugary foods is essential to prevent Kapha-related imbalances and maintain energy levels.

Daily Routine for Longevity

Ayurvedic principles stress the importance of a consistent daily routine, known as **Dinacharya**, to promote vitality, balance, and longevity. Adhering to a routine that supports the body's natural rhythms helps maintain physical, mental, and emotional well-being as we age.

- **Early to Bed, Early to Rise**: Ayurveda recommends going to bed by **10 PM** and waking up early to align with the body's circadian rhythms. Adequate sleep helps rejuvenate the body, maintain mental clarity, and balance hormones, supporting healthy aging.
- **Exercise**: Regular physical activity, tailored to one's doshic constitution, is essential for maintaining strength, flexibility, and energy levels. Vata types benefit from gentle exercises like walking or yoga, while Pitta types may thrive with moderate cardio, and Kapha types can benefit from more vigorous exercise to keep their energy levels high.
- **Self-Massage (Abhyanga)**: Regular self-massage with warm oils is a key Ayurvedic practice for rejuvenation. **Abhyanga** helps improve circulation, reduce stiffness, and calm the nervous system. Vata types should use **sesame oil**, while **coconut oil** is best for Pitta, and **mustard oil** can help stimulate circulation for Kapha.

Stress Management and Mental Health

Managing stress is critical for slowing the aging process. Chronic stress can lead to premature aging, cognitive decline, and imbalances in the body's doshas. Ayurvedic practices such as meditation, breathing exercises, and yoga are essential tools for maintaining mental health and emotional balance.

- **Pranayama** (breathing exercises) helps reduce mental agitation and calm the nervous system, promoting both mental clarity and emotional stability.
- **Meditation** helps cultivate inner peace, focus, and emotional resilience, which are key for healthy aging. Regular mindfulness practice also supports healthy brain function and reduces the harmful effects of stress.
- **Yoga** helps maintain flexibility, strength, and balance, while also calming the mind. Yoga promotes the circulation of energy throughout the body and aids in detoxification, which helps maintain youthfulness.

Skin and Hair Care for Aging Gracefully

In Ayurveda, the skin and hair are considered a reflection of the body's overall health. As we age, skin care focuses on hydration, nourishment, and supporting the body's detoxification processes.

- **Ghee**: **Ghee** is used topically to hydrate and rejuvenate dry, aging skin. It provides deep nourishment and helps retain moisture, preventing wrinkles and fine lines.
- **Turmeric and Aloe Vera**: **Turmeric** has antioxidant and anti-inflammatory properties that help reduce wrinkles, protect against sun damage, and rejuvenate the skin. **Aloe vera** helps soothe and hydrate dry or aging skin, promoting elasticity and preventing sagging.

For hair care, Ayurvedic remedies like **Bhringraj**, **Amla**, and **Shikakai** promote healthy hair growth, prevent graying, and maintain shine. Regular use of **herbal oils** and gentle hair treatments helps preserve hair health and prevent hair loss.

Ayurveda offers a comprehensive and balanced approach to aging, focusing on harmony between the body, mind, and spirit. Through proper diet, rejuvenating herbs, daily routines, stress management, and self-care practices, Ayurveda provides tools to age gracefully and maintain vitality well into later years. The key to healthy aging in Ayurveda lies not in fighting the passage of time but in understanding the body's natural cycles and nurturing it with balance, nourishment, and care. With these principles, aging becomes an opportunity to embrace vitality, wisdom, and well-being.

Ayurvedic Approach to Aging

In Ayurveda, aging is viewed as a natural process of transformation rather than a decline. This ancient system of medicine emphasizes the importance of maintaining balance and harmony within the body, mind, and spirit to age gracefully and preserve vitality. Ayurveda offers holistic solutions that focus not only on external treatments but also on internal health, promoting longevity through the balance of the doshas, digestion, lifestyle, and rejuvenating practices. Rather than fighting aging, Ayurveda encourages individuals to embrace it with a sense of vitality, wisdom, and harmony, recognizing that the aging process can be a time of personal growth and inner peace.

Doshas and Aging

According to Ayurveda, aging is directly related to the balance of the three doshas—**Vata**, **Pitta**, and **Kapha**—and their influence on the body's physical and mental state. As we age, the doshas shift, and these changes can affect the way we experience aging.

- **Vata**: Vata is associated with movement, dryness, and change. As Vata naturally increases with age, it can lead to dryness of the skin, hair, and joints. Vata imbalance can cause symptoms such as wrinkles, hair thinning, and arthritis. To counteract this, Ayurveda suggests nourishing, hydrating practices and grounding lifestyle routines to balance the increasing dryness and instability associated with Vata.
- **Pitta**: Pitta governs transformation, heat, and metabolism. In the aging process, excess Pitta can lead to inflammation, skin rashes, premature graying, and digestive disturbances. Cooling and soothing treatments that calm the heat within the body are essential for aging individuals with a predominant Pitta dosha.
- **Kapha**: Kapha governs structure, stability, and lubrication. While Kapha brings strength and endurance, an imbalance of this dosha during aging can lead to sluggishness, weight gain, and emotional stagnation. Stimulating and detoxifying practices are recommended to maintain Kapha balance and prevent excess accumulation in the body, helping to preserve energy and youthful vitality.

Agni and Ama in Aging

In Ayurveda, **Agni** (digestive fire) plays a crucial role in the aging process. A strong Agni promotes proper digestion, nutrient absorption, and toxin elimination, all of which contribute to healthy aging. When Agni weakens over time, it can lead to the buildup of **Ama** (toxins), which accelerates the aging process and contributes to disease.

To maintain youthfulness, Ayurveda encourages:

- **Maintaining a strong Agni** by eating warm, fresh, and easily digestible foods, avoiding overeating or consuming heavy, processed foods.
- **Detoxification** practices like **Panchakarma**, a series of therapeutic treatments that cleanse the body of accumulated toxins, improve digestion, and restore balance.

Rasayana (Rejuvenation) Therapy

A key Ayurvedic approach to slowing the aging process is **Rasayana** therapy, which focuses on rejuvenation and strengthening the body's tissues, boosting immunity, and improving longevity. Rasayana promotes the balance of the doshas and enhances Ojas, the vital energy that sustains life.

- **Herbs for Rejuvenation**: Ayurveda uses several rejuvenating herbs to slow aging, boost vitality, and improve overall health. Common herbs include **Amalaki** (Indian gooseberry), which is rich in antioxidants and vitamin C, **Brahmi**, known for its ability to calm the mind and improve mental clarity, and **Ashwagandha**, an adaptogen that combats stress and promotes strength.
- **Diet and Lifestyle**: A balanced diet rich in fresh, seasonal fruits and vegetables, whole grains, and healthy fats supports Rasayana therapy. Regular exercise, adequate sleep, and mindful living also play a significant role in maintaining vitality and slowing the aging process.

Anti-Aging Practices and Ayurvedic Treatments

Ayurveda promotes several daily practices and treatments to slow the physical and mental effects of aging. These practices focus on nourishment, rejuvenation, and detoxification.

1. **Abhyanga (Self-Massage)**: Abhyanga, the practice of self-massage with warm oils, is one of Ayurveda's most important rejuvenating techniques. It enhances circulation, reduces stiffness, and nourishes the skin. For Vata imbalances, **sesame oil** is often used for its grounding and warming properties, while **coconut oil** is recommended for Pitta types to soothe inflammation. **Mustard oil** is used for Kapha types to stimulate circulation and detoxify the body.
2. **Yoga and Pranayama**: Regular **yoga** is essential for maintaining flexibility, strength, and vitality as we age. Certain postures, such as **Tadasana** (Mountain Pose) and **Savasana** (Corpse Pose), help reduce stress, improve circulation, and encourage relaxation. **Pranayama** (breathing exercises), such as **Nadi Shodhana**

(alternate nostril breathing), help balance the nervous system, improve oxygen flow, and rejuvenate the body.
3. **Meditation**: Meditation is a crucial practice for maintaining mental clarity and emotional stability as we age. **Mindfulness meditation** and **loving-kindness meditation** help reduce stress, cultivate inner peace, and prevent the mental agitation that often accompanies aging. By fostering a calm mind, these practices support overall health and longevity.
4. **Herbal and Dietary Support**: In addition to Rasayana herbs, Ayurveda encourages the use of specific dietary practices to support aging. Consuming **ghee**, a rich source of healthy fats, helps nourish the tissues, lubricate joints, and enhance memory. **Turmeric**, with its anti-inflammatory properties, helps reduce the signs of aging, protect the skin, and maintain joint health. **Honey**, when consumed in moderation, nourishes the skin and promotes vitality.

Emotional and Mental Balance

In Ayurveda, aging is not just a physical process—it also involves mental and emotional transformation. Maintaining emotional balance and mental clarity is essential for graceful aging.

- **Emotional Well-Being**: Ayurveda recognizes that unresolved emotions, stress, and mental tension can manifest physically, accelerating the aging process. Practices like **journaling**, **therapy**, and spending time in nature are recommended to help release emotional blockages and maintain a peaceful mind.
- **Mental Clarity**: As we age, cognitive function may decline. Ayurveda promotes the use of **Brahmi** and **Ashwagandha** to improve memory, reduce mental fatigue, and support overall cognitive health.

Healthy Aging and the Environment

Living in harmony with nature and aligning your daily habits with natural rhythms plays a significant role in maintaining health and vitality as you age. Ayurveda recommends:

- **Aligning with the seasons**: Eating seasonal foods, adjusting routines to suit the environment, and making lifestyle changes according to the seasons can help balance the doshas and prevent premature aging.
- **Being present**: Living mindfully and embracing a lifestyle that encourages relaxation, creativity, and personal growth can promote happiness, vitality, and inner peace as you age.

In Ayurveda, aging is viewed as a natural progression of life that can be embraced with vitality, strength, and balance. By focusing on nourishing the body and mind, practicing rejuvenating therapies, and maintaining a balanced lifestyle, Ayurveda offers tools to slow the aging process and promote longevity. Aging gracefully in Ayurveda involves cultivating harmony between the internal and external, allowing individuals to thrive at every stage of life. Through proper self-care, stress management, and a balanced diet, Ayurveda enables individuals to enjoy health, vitality, and wisdom as they grow older.

Healthy Aging with Ayurveda

In Ayurveda, healthy aging is about maintaining balance in the body, mind, and spirit as one progresses through the different stages of life. Aging is viewed not as a decline but as a natural process that can be gracefully managed with the right practices, diet, and lifestyle. Ayurveda believes that the key to aging well lies in harmonizing the three doshas—**Vata**, **Pitta**, and **Kapha**—and addressing the unique needs of the body as it ages. By focusing on rejuvenation, nourishment, and stress management, Ayurveda offers a holistic approach to ensuring vitality, mental clarity, and emotional well-being throughout the aging process.

The Role of Doshas in Aging

Each dosha impacts the aging process in different ways, and an imbalance in any of them can accelerate the effects of aging. Ayurveda teaches that the proper balance of the doshas throughout life is essential to aging healthily.

- **Vata**: As Vata increases with age, it can lead to dryness in the skin, joints, and hair, as well as to mental restlessness and anxiety. When Vata is in balance, it promotes creativity, vitality, and flexibility. However, as Vata tends to increase with age, it can lead to conditions like joint pain, brittle bones, and cognitive decline. To manage Vata imbalances, Ayurveda recommends grounding practices, nourishing foods, and hydration to maintain softness in the skin and joints and clarity in the mind.
- **Pitta**: Pitta governs transformation and metabolism and is associated with heat. As people age, excess Pitta can lead to inflammation, digestive issues, and premature graying of hair. It can also contribute to skin problems like acne or rashes. Cooling foods, stress-reduction techniques, and anti-inflammatory herbs are essential for managing Pitta as one ages. Properly balancing Pitta helps maintain smooth skin, healthy digestion, and overall vitality.
- **Kapha**: Kapha provides structure and stability and is associated with the body's lubrication and growth. As Kapha energy becomes more pronounced in aging, it can lead to weight gain, sluggishness, and fluid retention. It may also cause emotional stagnation or a sense of heaviness. To maintain balance, Kapha types should engage in more stimulating activities, eat lighter, detoxifying foods, and focus on mental clarity to prevent emotional stagnation.

Diet and Nutrition for Healthy Aging

In Ayurveda, food is considered medicine, and the right diet is key to preventing premature aging and supporting vitality as we grow older. Proper digestion (**Agni**) is central to the Ayurvedic approach, as a strong Agni allows the body to absorb nutrients efficiently and eliminate toxins (**Ama**). Aging requires special attention to diet that promotes longevity, nourishes the body's tissues, and strengthens the digestive fire.

- **For Vata**: Vata types benefit from warm, moist, and grounding foods that combat dryness and imbalance. **Whole grains**, **cooked vegetables**, **ghee**, and **healthy fats** like **avocados** and **nuts** are essential to keeping the skin hydrated and preventing aging. Vata types should avoid cold, raw foods, excessive caffeine, and alcohol, as they can increase dryness and contribute to early aging signs like wrinkles and joint discomfort.
- **For Pitta**: Cooling foods help balance Pitta's heat and prevent premature aging related to inflammation. **Leafy greens**, **cucumbers**, **coconut**, **dairy**, and **fresh fruits** are ideal for cooling and soothing the skin. Avoiding spicy, greasy, or acidic foods helps maintain smooth skin, healthy digestion, and emotional balance. **Turmeric**, **mint**, and **fennel** are also recommended for their anti-inflammatory properties.
- **For Kapha**: To avoid weight gain and sluggishness, Kapha types should opt for lighter foods that promote circulation and metabolism. **Spicy foods**, **legumes**, **bitter greens**, and **cruciferous vegetables** like **broccoli** and **cauliflower** are beneficial for detoxifying and stimulating energy. Kapha types should avoid heavy, sweet, and oily foods, as these contribute to weight gain and emotional stagnation, which can accelerate aging.

Rejuvenation and Rasayana Therapy

Rasayana, the Ayurvedic science of rejuvenation, offers a set of practices and therapies designed to promote longevity, improve vitality, and slow the aging process. Rasayana focuses on nourishing the tissues, strengthening the immune system, and supporting the body's natural detoxification processes. Some of the key components of Rasayana therapy include:

- **Herbal Remedies**: Herbs like **Amalaki** (Indian gooseberry), **Brahmi**, **Ashwagandha**, and **Shatavari** are commonly used in Rasayana therapy. **Amalaki**, rich in antioxidants and vitamin C, strengthens the immune system and improves skin health, preventing premature wrinkles and sagging. **Brahmi** enhances cognitive function, reduces stress, and supports mental clarity, while **Ashwagandha** combats stress and promotes physical strength and vitality.
- **Ghee**: **Ghee**, a clarified butter, is considered one of the most important rejuvenating foods in Ayurveda. It nourishes tissues, lubricates joints, and

supports mental clarity. **Ghee** is also believed to improve digestion and strengthen the immune system, promoting overall health and vitality.
- **Panchakarma**: Panchakarma is a detoxification treatment that helps cleanse the body of toxins (**Ama**) and restore balance. This process helps rejuvenate the body by removing waste and impurities, allowing the tissues to be nourished and revitalized. Regular detoxification is recommended for healthy aging to maintain a strong **Agni** and prevent the accumulation of toxins that accelerate aging.

Daily Routines for Aging Gracefully

A consistent, balanced daily routine (**Dinacharya**) is essential for slowing down the aging process and promoting overall health. Ayurveda recommends simple daily practices to support healthy aging.

- **Self-massage (Abhyanga)**: Regular self-massage with warm oils helps improve circulation, reduce stress, and nourish the skin. It promotes relaxation, improves joint flexibility, and strengthens tissues, which is especially important as we age. For Vata types, **sesame oil** is ideal for its grounding properties, while **coconut oil** is cooling for Pitta, and **mustard oil** is stimulating for Kapha.
- **Exercise**: Regular physical activity is crucial for maintaining strength, flexibility, and vitality. Yoga, walking, or swimming are ideal for aging individuals, as they promote circulation, improve joint health, and maintain muscle tone. Regular movement also helps reduce stress, prevent weight gain, and balance the doshas.
- **Adequate Rest**: Ayurveda stresses the importance of sleep for rejuvenation. Going to bed early, ideally before **10 PM**, allows the body to rest and repair itself. A consistent sleep schedule helps maintain hormonal balance, reduces stress, and supports mental clarity.
- **Mindfulness Practices**: Meditation, breathing exercises (**Pranayama**), and stress-management techniques are essential for maintaining emotional well-being. These practices help cultivate inner peace, reduce mental agitation, and promote emotional resilience—key components of graceful aging.

The Role of Mental and Emotional Health

Ayurveda recognizes that mental and emotional balance is just as important as physical health in the aging process. The mind can influence the body's health, and unresolved emotional stress can lead to physical ailments and accelerate aging. Practices like **meditation**, **journaling**, and **mindfulness** are essential for managing emotional stress and fostering mental clarity. Cultivating joy, purpose, and positive emotions helps enhance **Ojas** and promote a youthful outlook on life.

Ayurveda offers a comprehensive and holistic approach to healthy aging, focusing on balance, nourishment, rejuvenation, and vitality. By understanding the role of the doshas, maintaining strong **Agni**, and following a lifestyle that includes proper diet, daily routines, rejuvenating therapies, and stress management, individuals can age gracefully and enjoy a long, healthy life. Ayurveda teaches that aging is not something to fear but an opportunity to deepen wisdom, embrace change, and enhance one's connection to life. Through the principles of Ayurveda, individuals can maintain vitality, mental clarity, and emotional well-being throughout the aging process.

Ayurvedic Herbs for Longevity

In Ayurveda, longevity is not simply about living longer but about maintaining vitality, strength, and balance throughout life. Achieving a long, healthy life is seen as the result of nourishing the body, mind, and spirit, supported by proper lifestyle, diet, and natural remedies. Ayurvedic herbs play a crucial role in promoting longevity by enhancing the body's natural ability to rejuvenate, detoxify, and balance the doshas. These herbs are carefully chosen to strengthen the immune system, enhance vitality, and reduce the effects of aging. Below are some of the most potent herbs used in Ayurveda for promoting longevity.

1. Ashwagandha (Withania somnifera)

Often referred to as the "king of herbs" in Ayurveda, **Ashwagandha** is an adaptogen that helps the body cope with stress, increase energy, and support overall vitality. It is widely used for its rejuvenating and anti-aging properties. Ashwagandha helps reduce cortisol levels, which are elevated during stress, and supports the adrenal glands, which can weaken with age. It also promotes muscle strength, cognitive function, and a sense of calm, making it an excellent herb for maintaining vitality as one ages.

2. Amalaki (Emblica officinalis)

Amalaki, or Indian gooseberry, is considered one of the most powerful rejuvenating herbs in Ayurveda. Rich in vitamin C, antioxidants, and essential fatty acids, Amalaki helps boost immunity, promote skin health, and slow down the aging process. It enhances digestion, reduces inflammation, and detoxifies the body by eliminating harmful free radicals. Regular use of Amalaki helps support longevity by strengthening the immune system and improving the overall vitality of the body.

3. Shatavari (Asparagus racemosus)

Shatavari is particularly beneficial for maintaining vitality in both men and women as they age. Known for its ability to nourish and rejuvenate, it is often called the "queen of herbs" in Ayurvedic medicine. Shatavari supports the reproductive system, balances hormones, and promotes digestion. Its adaptogenic properties help manage stress, and it strengthens the immune system, contributing to overall longevity. Shatavari is especially beneficial for older adults as it helps combat fatigue, restore energy levels, and maintain youthful vitality.

4. Brahmi (Bacopa monnieri)

Brahmi is a powerful herb for cognitive longevity. It is known for its ability to enhance mental clarity, improve memory, and reduce anxiety. Brahmi supports the nervous system by nourishing the brain and promoting mental agility. Its antioxidant properties help protect the brain from age-related cognitive decline, such as memory loss and mental fatigue. By improving cognitive function and reducing stress, Brahmi is an excellent herb for those seeking to preserve mental sharpness well into their later years.

5. Turmeric (Curcuma longa)

Turmeric is a well-known herb for its anti-inflammatory and antioxidant properties. The active compound in turmeric, **curcumin**, has been extensively studied for its ability to fight free radicals, reduce inflammation, and promote joint health. Regular consumption of turmeric helps slow the aging process by protecting the cells from oxidative damage, reducing the risk of chronic diseases, and improving skin health. Turmeric is also beneficial for the liver, promoting detoxification and supporting digestive health, both of which are crucial for maintaining vitality and longevity.

6. Ginger (Zingiber officinale)

Ginger is another herb with remarkable rejuvenating properties. It is known for its ability to stimulate digestion, improve circulation, and reduce inflammation. Ginger is also a potent antioxidant, helping to neutralize free radicals and protect against age-related degeneration. By enhancing blood flow and supporting detoxification, ginger promotes healthy aging and vitality. It also aids in reducing muscle stiffness, improving joint health, and supporting the immune system, making it a versatile herb for longevity.

7. Gokshura (Tribulus terrestris)

Gokshura is a rejuvenating herb that enhances vitality, strength, and endurance. It is commonly used to support the reproductive system and improve overall stamina, particularly in aging individuals. Gokshura is known for its ability to boost energy levels, support kidney function, and improve circulation. It also promotes healthy hormone levels, making it beneficial for managing the physical effects of aging, including low energy, decreased libido, and reduced muscle mass.

8. Holy Basil (Tulsi) (Ocimum sanctum)

Known as **Tulsi**, Holy Basil is revered in Ayurveda for its ability to promote longevity by reducing stress and boosting immunity. Tulsi is considered a sacred herb that enhances both physical and mental well-being. It is highly effective in combating stress, improving respiratory function, and promoting detoxification. The adaptogenic properties of Tulsi help the body adapt to various stresses, while its anti-inflammatory and antioxidant properties protect the body from age-related degeneration.

9. Gotu Kola (Centella Asiatica)

Gotu Kola, known as **Brahmi** in some parts of India, is an herb that promotes longevity through its cognitive benefits and its ability to support the skin. It is traditionally used to improve memory, reduce anxiety, and support healthy aging by enhancing circulation. Gotu Kola is also known for promoting collagen production in the skin, improving elasticity, and reducing wrinkles. Its ability to rejuvenate tissues and improve blood flow makes it an excellent herb for supporting overall vitality and longevity.

10. Saffron (Crocus sativus)

Saffron is a potent herb used in Ayurveda for its anti-aging and skin-rejuvenating properties. Rich in antioxidants, saffron helps combat free radicals that contribute to the aging process. It improves circulation, enhances skin tone, and promotes a glowing complexion. Saffron also has mood-enhancing properties, helping to reduce stress and anxiety, which is vital for healthy aging. Its ability to promote mental clarity and reduce inflammation makes it a valuable herb for longevity.

11. Ashitaba (Angelica Keiskei)

Native to Japan but also used in Ayurvedic medicine, **Ashitaba** is known for its powerful rejuvenating effects. It is rich in antioxidants, vitamins, and minerals that help support the immune system and promote cellular regeneration. Ashitaba is believed to enhance longevity by improving the body's ability to repair damaged cells, reduce inflammation, and prevent chronic diseases. Its antioxidant-rich profile helps protect against oxidative stress, which is a major factor in the aging process.

12. Moringa (Moringa oleifera)

Moringa is often called the "tree of life" due to its impressive nutritional profile. It contains a wide range of vitamins, minerals, antioxidants, and amino acids that support overall health and longevity. Moringa helps reduce inflammation, improve skin health, boost energy, and support brain function. It is also beneficial for maintaining healthy cholesterol levels, blood sugar, and liver function, all of which contribute to healthy aging.

Ayurvedic herbs are central to maintaining vitality and slowing the aging process by nurturing the body from within. These herbs, when used in combination with a balanced diet, healthy lifestyle, and mindful practices, can significantly enhance longevity and well-being. Whether you are looking to improve cognitive function, reduce inflammation, enhance energy, or rejuvenate your skin, these powerful herbs offer natural, holistic support for aging gracefully and maintaining health throughout the years.

Ayurvedic Treatments and Therapies

In Ayurveda, treatments and therapies are designed to restore balance and harmony within the body, mind, and spirit. The core philosophy of Ayurveda is that health is a reflection of the body's ability to maintain equilibrium between the three doshas—**Vata**, **Pitta**, and **Kapha**—as well as between the physical and emotional aspects of life. Ayurvedic treatments aim to promote wellness by addressing the root causes of imbalances and supporting the body's natural healing abilities. These therapies include a combination of diet, herbs, detoxification, lifestyle practices, and physical treatments that work together to restore health and vitality.

Panchakarma: The Ultimate Detoxification Therapy

One of the most well-known Ayurvedic therapies is **Panchakarma**, a comprehensive detoxification treatment designed to cleanse the body of toxins (**Ama**) and restore balance to the doshas. Panchakarma is typically recommended for those dealing with chronic health conditions or seeking a deep cleanse to rejuvenate the body. The therapy consists of five main procedures:

1. **Vamana (Emesis Therapy)**: Induces controlled vomiting to eliminate toxins and cleanse the upper digestive system, particularly helpful for Pitta imbalances.
2. **Virechana (Purgation Therapy)**: Involves the use of herbal laxatives to remove toxins from the lower digestive tract, typically beneficial for Pitta imbalances.
3. **Basti (Enema Therapy)**: Uses herbal oils or decoctions to cleanse the colon, benefiting Vata imbalances by hydrating and soothing the digestive system.
4. **Nasya (Nasal Therapy)**: The application of herbal oils or powders to the nasal passages to clear sinus congestion, enhance mental clarity, and detoxify the respiratory system.
5. **Raktamokshana (Bloodletting Therapy)**: Used to cleanse the blood, this therapy is particularly helpful in cases of skin conditions and inflammation.

Panchakarma helps detoxify the body, balance the doshas, improve digestion, enhance energy levels, and promote long-term health.

Shirodhara: Healing Through Oil

Shirodhara is a deeply relaxing Ayurvedic therapy that involves pouring a steady stream of warm, medicated oil onto the forehead, specifically targeting the **third eye** area (the space between the eyebrows). The oil is typically infused with herbs like **Brahmi** or **Jatamansi**, which help soothe the mind, calm the nervous system, and promote mental clarity. This therapy is widely used to treat conditions like anxiety, insomnia, stress, and mental fatigue. By stimulating the **Ajna chakra**, Shirodhara also helps to improve concentration and emotional stability, offering both physical and mental rejuvenation.

Abhyanga: Ayurvedic Massage for Rejuvenation

Abhyanga, or self-massage with warm, medicated oils, is a cornerstone of Ayurvedic therapy. It involves massaging the body with oils that are chosen according to the individual's dosha type. For example, **sesame oil** is often recommended for Vata types to promote grounding and hydration, while **coconut oil** is used for Pitta types to cool and calm the body. The benefits of Abhyanga are numerous—it improves circulation, detoxifies the body, nourishes the skin, promotes relaxation, and enhances the flow of energy (prana) throughout the body. Regular use of Abhyanga is known to slow down the aging process, reduce stress, improve joint mobility, and support overall vitality.

Swedana: Herbal Steam Therapy

Swedana, or herbal steam therapy, is often used as a complementary treatment to other Ayurvedic therapies like **Panchakarma**. During this treatment, the body is exposed to steam infused with herbal extracts, such as **ginger**, **turmeric**, or **eucalyptus**, which help open the pores, promote sweating, and facilitate the release of toxins from the body. Swedana enhances circulation, boosts the immune system, and promotes deep relaxation. It is particularly effective in managing conditions like joint pain, muscle stiffness, respiratory issues, and skin disorders.

Ayurvedic Diet and Nutrition

Ayurveda places great emphasis on the role of diet in maintaining health and treating illness. The Ayurvedic approach to nutrition involves eating foods that are tailored to the individual's dosha, season, and current state of health. A balanced diet supports digestion, enhances energy levels, and prevents the accumulation of toxins in the body.

- **For Vata**: A diet rich in warm, moist, and grounding foods is recommended. This includes **whole grains**, **root vegetables**, **ghee**, and **nuts** to hydrate and nourish the body, especially in the colder months.
- **For Pitta**: Cooling foods like **leafy greens**, **cucumbers**, and **coconut** help soothe Pitta's fiery nature. Dairy, fresh fruits, and moderate amounts of grains are ideal for maintaining balance.
- **For Kapha**: Light, stimulating foods such as **spices** (ginger, black pepper), **legumes**, and **cruciferous vegetables** help keep Kapha in check, especially for those prone to weight gain or lethargy.

Ayurveda also advocates mindful eating, which includes eating in a peaceful environment, chewing food thoroughly, and eating at regular intervals to support digestion (**Agni**).

Ayurvedic Herbs for Health and Healing

Ayurvedic herbs are used to address a wide range of health concerns, from chronic conditions to general wellness. Herbs like **Ashwagandha**, **Turmeric**, **Brahmi**, **Neem**, and **Ginger** have been used for centuries to promote health, strengthen the immune system, reduce inflammation, and balance the doshas. These herbs are often used in the form of teas, powders, or oils, and they are customized to meet the specific health needs of the individual.

- **Ashwagandha** is an adaptogen known for its ability to reduce stress, improve energy levels, and enhance vitality.
- **Turmeric** is a powerful anti-inflammatory herb used to support joint health, skin healing, and digestive function.
- **Brahmi** is used for mental clarity, stress reduction, and cognitive enhancement.
- **Neem** is known for its detoxifying and antibacterial properties, used to cleanse the blood and improve skin health.

Rasayana Therapy: Rejuvenation for Longevity

Rasayana refers to Ayurvedic therapies focused on rejuvenating and nourishing the tissues. It helps preserve and improve strength, vitality, and immunity. Rasayana therapies include specific herbs, rejuvenative practices, and lifestyle modifications designed to prolong life, enhance mental clarity, and maintain a youthful appearance. Common Rasayana herbs include **Amalaki**, **Brahmi**, and **Shatavari**, which are considered potent rejuvenators that support longevity and overall health. Rasayana not only enhances physical health but also promotes mental and emotional well-being, helping to achieve balance in all aspects of life.

Yoga and Pranayama: Energizing the Body and Mind

Yoga and **Pranayama** (breathing exercises) are essential components of Ayurvedic healing, designed to harmonize the body, mind, and spirit. Regular practice of yoga enhances flexibility, improves circulation, and supports digestion. Breathing exercises help manage stress, improve oxygen flow to the body, and detoxify the system. Together, these practices rejuvenate the body, increase energy, and promote mental clarity. Yoga also helps maintain strength, prevent muscle stiffness, and improve posture as the body ages.

Lifestyle Practices for Health and Balance

Ayurveda emphasizes the importance of a consistent daily routine (**Dinacharya**) to maintain health and prevent illness. Following a daily routine that aligns with the body's natural circadian rhythms is essential for longevity. This includes waking up early, practicing self-massage, engaging in regular exercise, eating meals at regular intervals, and ensuring adequate rest. Ayurveda also recommends mindfulness practices such as meditation, which help promote emotional stability, reduce stress, and enhance overall well-being.

Ayurvedic treatments and therapies offer a comprehensive, holistic approach to health and wellness. By focusing on detoxification, rejuvenation, personalized nutrition, herbal remedies, and physical therapies, Ayurveda supports not only the healing of existing conditions but also the promotion of long-term vitality and balance. These therapies address the root causes of imbalances, restore harmony within the body, and help individuals live longer, healthier, and more fulfilling lives.

Panchakarma - The Five Purification Procedures

In Ayurveda, **Panchakarma** is a highly effective and comprehensive detoxification therapy designed to cleanse the body of toxins (**Ama**) and restore balance to the doshas (Vata, Pitta, and Kapha). The term "Panchakarma" literally means "five actions" or "five therapies," which refers to the five purification procedures used to cleanse the body on both a physical and mental level. These therapies are individualized to suit the person's doshic constitution and health concerns, and they work together to rejuvenate the body, strengthen immunity, and restore optimal health. Panchakarma is often used for those seeking to address chronic health conditions or for preventive care, providing a holistic approach to wellness.

1. Vamana (Therapeutic Vomiting)

Vamana is the first of the five procedures and involves induced vomiting to eliminate excess mucus and toxins accumulated in the upper digestive system, primarily affecting the stomach and lungs. This procedure is particularly beneficial for individuals with **Kapha** imbalances, which manifest as excess mucous, congestion, or respiratory conditions like asthma or bronchitis.

The process begins with a preparatory phase, involving the administration of herbal oils or ghee to lubricate the body and soften the toxins. This is followed by the consumption of a medicated drink that induces vomiting, allowing the body to expel toxins and excess fluids. Vamana helps to clear the respiratory tract, relieve congestion, improve digestion, and reduce feelings of heaviness. It's especially effective in treating conditions related to chronic coughs, obesity, and metabolic disorders.

2. Virechana (Purgation Therapy)

Virechana, or purgation therapy, is used to cleanse the lower digestive tract, particularly the intestines, by eliminating excess **Pitta** (heat, fire, and transformation). This therapy is beneficial for individuals suffering from conditions related to Pitta imbalances, such as inflammatory skin diseases, acidity, jaundice, or digestive disturbances like diarrhea or irritable bowel syndrome (IBS).

Virechana is typically performed after the body has been prepared with an initial period of oiling and sweating, allowing the toxins to loosen and move towards the digestive tract. After this preparatory stage, a mixture of medicinal herbs and natural laxatives is given to induce a controlled purging of the bowels. This process helps cleanse the liver, gall bladder, and intestines, expelling toxic waste and balancing the Pitta dosha. It is a powerful method for improving digestive health and alleviating conditions related to excess bile or heat in the body.

3. Basti (Enema Therapy)

Basti is one of the most important and effective treatments in Panchakarma for balancing **Vata** dosha, which governs the movement and function of the body. The therapy involves the administration of herbal oils, decoctions, or milk-based solutions through the rectum, providing deep cleansing for the colon and intestines. It is used to remove deep-seated toxins and rejuvenate the colon, promoting better digestion and absorption of nutrients.

Basti therapy is especially helpful for conditions related to Vata imbalances, such as constipation, back pain, arthritis, and neurological disorders. The therapy has a calming and balancing effect on the nervous system, aiding in the treatment of both physical and mental health conditions. There are different types of Basti, including **Anuvasana Basti** (using oil-based solutions) and **Niruha Basti** (using decoctions), each tailored to the individual's needs. Regular Basti treatments help in maintaining healthy bowel function, enhancing overall digestion, and supporting detoxification.

4. Nasya (Nasal Therapy)

Nasya involves the administration of herbal oils or powders through the nostrils, targeting the sinuses and respiratory system. This therapy is particularly effective for individuals suffering from conditions caused by an excess of **Kapha** or **Vata**, such as sinus congestion, allergies, headaches, or nasal blockages. Nasya helps to cleanse the upper respiratory tract, remove excess mucus, and clear the head and sinuses.

The therapy begins with a gentle massage of the head and neck to stimulate the sinuses, followed by the application of medicated oils or powders to the nasal passages. Nasya has the added benefit of improving mental clarity, alleviating stress, and enhancing cognitive function by promoting better oxygen flow to the brain. It is also beneficial for conditions such as migraines, chronic sinusitis, and sleep disorders. Nasya is known to rejuvenate the senses, promoting mental alertness and emotional stability.

5. Raktamokshana (Bloodletting Therapy)

Raktamokshana is an Ayurvedic therapy that involves the controlled removal of small quantities of blood from the body to detoxify the bloodstream and improve circulation. This therapy is especially useful for individuals with skin conditions such as acne, eczema, or psoriasis, as it helps purify the blood and reduce the inflammation and toxicity that contribute to these conditions.

Raktamokshana is performed using a variety of techniques, including **leech therapy**, **suction**, or **syringe**. The process is highly beneficial in treating conditions related to **Pitta** imbalances, such as inflammatory diseases, skin issues, and certain blood disorders. By removing excess heat and toxins from the blood, Raktamokshana promotes better skin health, reduces the risk of infections, and helps balance the body's internal environment.

Benefits of Panchakarma

The Panchakarma therapies offer numerous benefits, both immediate and long-term, for overall health and wellness. Some of the key advantages include:

1. **Detoxification**: Panchakarma clears the body of accumulated toxins, which helps prevent diseases, boosts immunity, and rejuvenates the body.
2. **Rejuvenation**: These therapies help rejuvenate the tissues, improve digestion, and restore balance to the doshas, leading to a more youthful appearance and increased energy levels.
3. **Stress Relief**: The process of detoxifying the body and calming the mind helps reduce stress, anxiety, and mental fatigue, leading to better emotional well-being.
4. **Improved Digestion**: Panchakarma therapies enhance **Agni** (digestive fire), improving metabolism, absorption, and elimination, which are key to maintaining overall health.
5. **Weight Management**: By cleansing the body of excess toxins and promoting better digestion, Panchakarma can help manage weight and support a healthy metabolism.
6. **Boosted Immunity**: Detoxification strengthens the immune system, making the body more resilient to illnesses and external toxins.

Panchakarma is a profound and holistic approach to detoxification, rejuvenation, and healing in Ayurveda. By utilizing the five purification procedures—Vamana, Virechana, Basti, Nasya, and Raktamokshana—Panchakarma works to restore balance to the body's doshas, cleanse internal systems, and promote overall wellness. This ancient therapy is highly effective in addressing a wide range of health conditions, enhancing vitality, and slowing down the aging process. Panchakarma provides deep cleansing, inner rejuvenation, and lasting health benefits when incorporated into a balanced lifestyle and wellness regimen.

Ayurvedic Massages and Their Benefits

In Ayurveda, massage is considered an essential therapeutic practice that helps restore balance and harmony within the body, mind, and spirit. Ayurvedic massages are designed to nourish the body, promote circulation, detoxify, and address the root causes of physical and mental imbalances. The practice uses warm, medicated oils that are selected based on an individual's dosha (Vata, Pitta, or Kapha), offering a personalized approach to healing. Ayurvedic massages not only improve physical health but also enhance emotional well-being and promote deep relaxation.

Abhyanga: The Classic Ayurvedic Self-Massage

One of the most well-known Ayurvedic massages is **Abhyanga**, which involves the application of warm, herbal oils to the body in a rhythmic, soothing manner. This practice is deeply nourishing, providing benefits such as improved circulation, reduced stress, and enhanced skin tone.

- **For Vata types**, **sesame oil** is commonly used to provide grounding and warmth, addressing dryness and reducing Vata imbalances like joint pain or anxiety.
- **For Pitta types**, **coconut oil** is preferred for its cooling properties, helping to calm inflammation, soothe irritated skin, and reduce the heat that Pitta types often experience.
- **For Kapha types**, **mustard oil** or **sesame oil** may be used to invigorate the body, stimulate circulation, and remove excess moisture and stagnation.

Abhyanga helps balance the doshas by enhancing the body's ability to detoxify and release toxins (Ama). Regular Abhyanga promotes relaxation, improves flexibility, strengthens muscles, and increases energy levels. It also calms the nervous system and has a rejuvenating effect, making it particularly beneficial for those dealing with stress or mental fatigue.

Shirodhara: Oil Therapy for the Mind

Shirodhara is a specialized form of Ayurvedic massage that focuses on the forehead, particularly on the **third eye** area, where a steady stream of warm, medicated oil is poured. This therapeutic oil treatment is designed to promote mental clarity, relieve stress, and calm the nervous system.

Shirodhara is highly beneficial for those dealing with anxiety, insomnia, and mental fatigue. It helps balance the **Vata** dosha and promotes deep relaxation. The soothing flow of oil stimulates the **Ajna chakra**, improving concentration and emotional well-being. This treatment is also known to relieve tension in the head, neck, and shoulders, reducing headaches and migraines.

Pinda Swedana: Herbal Bundle Therapy

Pinda Swedana is an Ayurvedic massage that uses warm herbal bundles to massage the body, especially areas affected by pain or stiffness. The bundles, filled with medicated herbs, are dipped in warm oils or decoctions, and then applied to the body through gentle, rhythmic strokes. This therapy is particularly effective for Vata imbalances, such as joint pain, muscle stiffness, or fatigue.

The heat and herbal infusion from the bundles help increase circulation, promote sweating, and release toxins from deep within the tissues. Pinda Swedana is highly beneficial for conditions like arthritis, sports injuries, and muscle strains, as it helps reduce pain, improve mobility, and soothe sore muscles. It also promotes relaxation and detoxification.

Udvartana: Dry Powder Massage

Udvartana is a unique Ayurvedic massage that involves the application of herbal powders, often mixed with oils, to the skin. The herbal powders are massaged into the body using an invigorating, upward stroke, helping to exfoliate the skin and stimulate the circulation of **lymphatic fluid**. This massage is especially effective for Kapha imbalances, such as excess weight, sluggish digestion, and cellulite.

The dry powder exfoliates the skin, improving texture and tone while promoting the detoxification of the skin's surface. The stimulating effect of Udvartana helps in fat breakdown and improves metabolism, which is beneficial for weight management. This massage also boosts circulation, reduces water retention, and invigorates the body, making it an excellent choice for those looking to rejuvenate and energize.

Marma Therapy: Targeting Energy Points

Marma therapy involves the gentle application of pressure on specific energy points, or **marma points**, throughout the body. These points are similar to acupressure points, and stimulating them helps balance the flow of vital energy (prana) in the body. Marma therapy is highly beneficial for reducing stress, improving mental clarity, and relieving chronic pain.

By focusing on marma points, the therapist helps remove blockages in the energy pathways, encouraging better circulation and the proper functioning of organs and tissues. Marma therapy is used to treat a variety of conditions, including digestive issues, headaches, and joint pain, as well as to enhance the body's overall vitality.

Benefits of Ayurvedic Massages

The therapeutic effects of Ayurvedic massages extend beyond relaxation, offering a wide range of physical, mental, and emotional benefits. Some of the key advantages include:

- **Detoxification**: Ayurvedic massages help stimulate the lymphatic system, promote sweating, and release toxins (Ama) from the body. This detoxification process cleanses the body and promotes overall health.
- **Stress Reduction**: The rhythmic movements and soothing effects of Ayurvedic oils help activate the parasympathetic nervous system, which reduces stress, promotes relaxation, and improves sleep quality.
- **Improved Circulation**: Massaging with warm oils enhances blood circulation, delivering nutrients to tissues and organs more efficiently, while also improving the skin's tone and elasticity.
- **Skin Health**: The nourishing oils used in Ayurvedic massages hydrate the skin, improve its texture, and reduce dryness, fine lines, and wrinkles. These treatments also stimulate the production of collagen, which promotes skin firmness and elasticity.
- **Pain Relief**: Ayurvedic massages, such as **Pinda Swedana** and **Abhyanga**, help alleviate muscle stiffness, joint pain, and inflammation. These therapies can provide relief for conditions such as arthritis, fibromyalgia, and muscle strain.
- **Improved Flexibility**: Regular Ayurvedic massage helps release tension in the muscles and joints, improving flexibility and range of motion, which is particularly beneficial for older adults or those experiencing joint discomfort.
- **Emotional Well-Being**: The calming effects of Ayurvedic massages not only promote physical health but also help improve mental clarity, reduce anxiety, and promote emotional stability. These therapies are especially beneficial for individuals dealing with stress or emotional imbalances.

Ayurvedic massages are a cornerstone of holistic health, offering a natural way to restore balance, improve circulation, and rejuvenate the body. With their ability to detoxify, relieve stress, and promote overall well-being, these therapies are invaluable tools for enhancing health and vitality. By choosing the right Ayurvedic massage for their specific needs, individuals can experience long-lasting benefits, from better skin and enhanced flexibility to improved mental clarity and emotional balance. Whether through soothing **Abhyanga**, invigorating **Udvartana**, or therapeutic **Shirodhara**, Ayurvedic massages provide a path to rejuvenation, vitality, and wellness.

Marma Therapy in Ayurveda

In Ayurveda, **Marma therapy** is a powerful healing technique that focuses on the stimulation of specific energy points in the body called **marma points**. These points are analogous to acupressure or acupuncture points and are believed to be key intersections where the body's vital energy (**prana**) flows. By applying gentle pressure to these marma points, Marma therapy aims to unblock energy pathways, restore balance to the doshas, and promote overall health and well-being. This technique is deeply rooted in Ayurvedic medicine, which emphasizes the interconnectedness of the body, mind, and spirit.

The Concept of Marma Points

Marma points are thought to be sensitive areas in the body where energy, blood vessels, muscles, tendons, and bones intersect. In Ayurveda, there are 107 primary marma points, each with its own significance and role in the body's energy system. These points are spread across the body, including areas like the head, neck, chest, back, arms, and legs. Each marma point is associated with specific organs and tissues, and stimulating these points can have profound therapeutic effects on both the physical and mental health of an individual.

The word "marma" comes from the Sanskrit term for "hidden" or "secret," reflecting the depth and complexity of the energy centers within the body. These points are considered gateways to the body's internal energy and healing potential, and when manipulated correctly, they can help activate the body's natural healing processes.

How Marma Therapy Works

Marma therapy works by applying direct pressure or a subtle massage technique to specific points on the body. This pressure can be applied with fingers, palms, or even special tools like marma sticks. The intention behind the therapy is to restore the flow of **prana** (life energy) that may be obstructed due to emotional, physical, or environmental stress.

When marma points are stimulated, they help to balance the doshas (Vata, Pitta, and Kapha) by releasing stored energy and facilitating the movement of prana through the body. This improves circulation, reduces tension, and enhances the body's ability to heal itself. In Ayurvedic practice, marma therapy is often combined with other treatments such as **Abhyanga** (self-massage), **Panchakarma** (detoxification therapies), and **meditation** for a more comprehensive approach to health.

Benefits of Marma Therapy

Marma therapy offers a wide range of physical, mental, and emotional benefits. Some of the most notable advantages include:

1. **Pain Relief**: Marma therapy is effective in relieving chronic pain, particularly in the joints, muscles, and connective tissues. By stimulating the marma points, tension is released, which reduces discomfort caused by conditions like arthritis, muscle spasms, and back pain.
2. **Improved Circulation**: The stimulation of marma points enhances blood flow throughout the body, improving oxygen delivery to tissues and organs. This supports detoxification and helps improve overall vitality.
3. **Stress Reduction**: Marma therapy calms the nervous system by releasing stored emotional and physical tension. It is especially helpful for reducing stress, anxiety, and emotional blockages. Regular marma therapy can create a deep sense of relaxation, contributing to better sleep and a more balanced emotional state.
4. **Enhanced Digestion**: Certain marma points are linked to the digestive system. Stimulating these points can help regulate metabolism, promote better digestion, and alleviate conditions such as bloating, indigestion, and constipation.
5. **Mental Clarity**: Marma therapy helps improve mental focus, concentration, and clarity. By unlocking energy in the body and mind, it clears mental fog and promotes emotional stability, reducing feelings of confusion or mental fatigue.
6. **Detoxification**: By stimulating energy flow, marma therapy promotes the release of toxins and waste products from the body. This detoxifying effect supports the immune system and improves skin health by reducing inflammation and acne.
7. **Improved Flexibility and Mobility**: The therapy works to release stiffness in the muscles and joints, increasing flexibility and range of motion. This is particularly beneficial for people who experience limited mobility or stiffness due to age or injury.

Marma Therapy for Emotional Healing

Beyond physical health, marma therapy also plays a significant role in emotional and psychological well-being. According to Ayurveda, unresolved emotions can become trapped in the body, leading to blockages in energy flow. These blockages manifest as physical ailments, mental health issues, or emotional disturbances.

Marma therapy addresses these emotional imbalances by unblocking stagnant energy, allowing emotions to be released in a healthy way. It can help heal emotional wounds, reduce stress-related emotional symptoms (like anxiety or irritability), and improve mental clarity. Marma therapy encourages mindfulness and self-awareness, helping individuals connect with their inner selves and achieve emotional balance.

Marma Points and Their Specific Benefits

Each marma point is associated with different functions in the body. Some of the key marma points include:

- **Ajna Marma (Third Eye)**: Located between the eyebrows, this point is associated with intuition, mental clarity, and emotional stability. Stimulating this point helps reduce stress, clear mental fog, and enhance spiritual awareness.
- **Sthapani Marma (Forehead)**: Situated on the forehead, this marma point is beneficial for enhancing cognitive function and improving memory. It is also helpful for reducing tension headaches and improving focus.
- **Hridaya Marma (Heart)**: Located in the chest area, the Hridaya point is associated with emotional well-being and heart health. Stimulating this point can help reduce anxiety, improve circulation, and promote a feeling of love and compassion.
- **Kshipra Marma (Neck)**: Situated on the neck, this point helps release tension in the shoulders and neck. It is beneficial for alleviating neck pain, improving flexibility, and enhancing respiratory function.
- **Knee Marma (Janu)**: The knee marma point is important for joint health. It helps with the release of tension in the knees, supports mobility, and alleviates conditions like arthritis.

How Marma Therapy is Performed

Marma therapy is typically administered by an experienced Ayurvedic practitioner who understands the specific marma points and their therapeutic effects. The therapist applies gentle pressure or subtle massage to the identified points, using oils or herbal pastes suited to the individual's dosha and health condition.

In some cases, marma therapy may involve the use of additional techniques such as **shirodhara** (oil pouring on the forehead), **nasya** (nasal therapy), or **abhyanga** (full-body massage) to enhance the effects of marma point stimulation.

Marma therapy is a powerful, yet gentle Ayurvedic treatment that addresses the body's energy system and enhances overall health. By focusing on specific energy points throughout the body, this therapy promotes detoxification, pain relief, emotional healing, and mental clarity. Regular Marma therapy sessions can help individuals achieve a state of balance, vitality, and well-being, contributing to improved physical, emotional, and spiritual health. Whether used for relaxation, healing, or rejuvenation, Marma therapy remains one of the most effective tools in Ayurvedic medicine.

Have Questions / Comments?

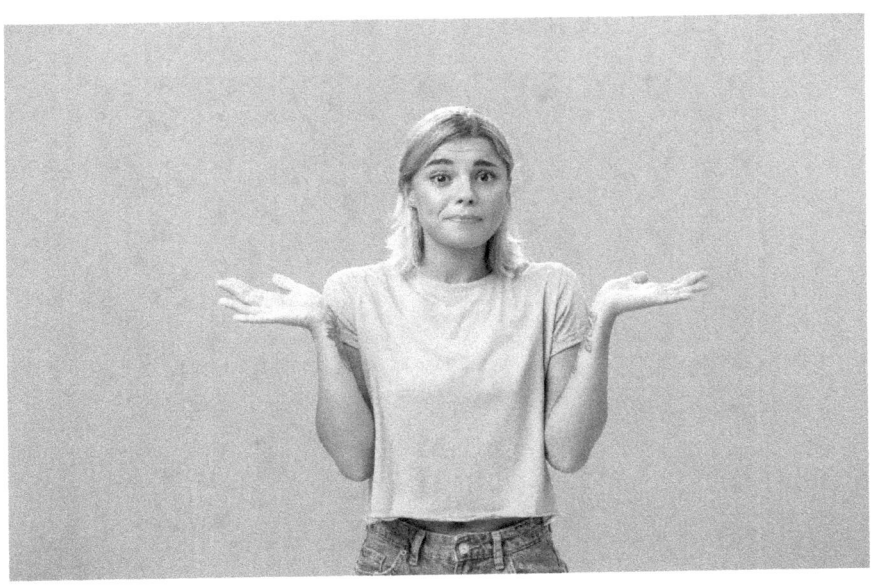

This book was designed to cover as much as possible but I know I have probably missed something, or some new amazing discovery that has just come out.

If you notice something missing or have a question that I failed to answer, please get in touch and let me know. If I can, I will email you an answer and also update the book so others can also benefit from it.

Thanks For Being Awesome :)

Submit Your Questions / Comments At:

https://questions.xspurts.com

Get Another Book Free

We love writing and have produced a huge number of books.

For being one of our amazing readers, we would love to offer you another book we have created, 100% free.

To claim this limited time special offer, simply go to the site below and enter your name and email address.

You will then receive one of my great books, direct to your email account, 100% free!

https://free.xspurts.com